Clinical Clues

A collection of EMS case studies

by

Paul Werfel, BA, NREMT-P

Clinical Clues

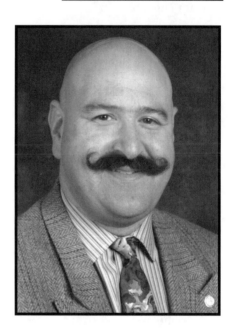

Published by:
Jems Communications, The Journal of Emergency Medical
Services

Publisher:
Jeff Berend

Editor: Keri Losavio

Cover Design and Production:
Janene Long-Forman
Lynn Papenhausen

ISBN 0-936174-15-3

Journal of Emergency Medical Services is published by:
Jems Communications
525 B. Street, Suite 1900
San Diego, CA 92101-4495
800/266-5367
www.jems.com

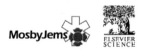

Printed and bound in the United States of America.

This book is dedicated to my family:

*My wife Karen, daughters
Emily Sarah and Molly Jane
and son Benjamin Alan.
You have shown me that with patience,
love and support, anything is possible*

Contents

5 Medical Emergencies

6 Geriatric Emergencies

7 Neurological Emergencies

8 Toxicological Emergencies

9 Environmental Emergencies

Foreword

I remember the hard work it took to complete my paramedic program requirements and be cleared to take my certification exam. I studied for weeks prior to the exam, reviewing blood types, indications and contraindications to drugs, cardiac rhythms and treatment algorithms. I felt prepared when I sat for my exam and was thrilled when notified that I had passed. I couldn't wait to complete my internship and become cleared to save the world.

When it came time for me to serve as the solo paramedic on an 1800–0600 shift one cold, winter evening, I wondered what challenges I would face. Would it be a respiratory arrest or a cardiac arrest? Would I be able to establish an IV on the patient?

When my pager went off for my first ALS case—a patient with chest pain in a local restaurant—I almost coded myself. I wondered if I would remember everything I had been taught. On scene, I soon realized that EMS encompasses far more than assessing and treating patients.

Restaurant customers were more concerned about how we were interfering with their meals than the man's wet, pasty skin and chest pain. There was no room to set up our radio, monitor and drug box next to the patient. And his long-sleeve shirt, sweater, vest and sport coat presented obstacles I had never encountered in my training, hospital rotations or field internship.

Assessment is one of the most important aspects of pre-hospital medicine. But assessment includes much more than the physical assessment of a patient. It also includes scene assessment, an assessment of the sincerity in the voices of patients and their family members and an assessment of the progress you and your partners are making in resolving each patient's problems.

During EMS educational programs, personnel receive quality lessons on all aspects of patient assessment and myriad medical, traumatic, environmental and psychological conditions. However, class time is limited. Instructors can't always present the bizarre things that can complicate field assessments, such as noisy restaurants, sour smells and intoxicated bystanders.

This book offers readers something that few other EMS books do—the opportunity to experience a host of different cases, each with its unique scenarios, facts and complications.

Paul Werfel has crafted educationally sound and professional EMS field stories that place you on scene with EMS personnel responding to real-world incidents that challenge you to think and educate you in the process. He has masterfully woven important scene circumstances and vital signs that deviate from the norm into case presentations that challenge the minds of newly certified EMS personnel and seasoned veterans.

Paul's extensive background as a field provider and educator has enabled him to educate and entertain readers with his cases. His writing style and sense of humor bring his cases alive and allow you to get involved in each patient assessment.

Most importantly, each case presents a different challenge that forces you to dig deep into your educational memory bank. If you recognize the patient's problem or can use the information presented to solve the patient puzzle, you get a sense of professional pride. If you can't, Paul's educational summary cues you into the circumstances and final patient outcome, educating you and arming you with important information to assist you with future cases.

A.J. Heightman, MPA, EMT-P
Editor
JEMS (Journal of Emergency Medical Services)
November 2002

Preface

If you take the time to look at the diplomas you received when you graduated from your EMS training course, you will see that most of them confer privileges and obligations to the graduate. EMS practitioners are truly privileged to be allowed into people's lives to erase their pain, offer a helping hand and, yes, even save a life now and then. Many of us do more public good in a week than most folks do in a lifetime.

Our obligations are to provide good, compassionate care to our patients. With a dynamic medicolegal landscape and new drugs, procedures and therapies being developed by the day, it is easy to see how our shoulders could bow under the pressure of our privileges and obligations.

Good solid education is the reason we have been able to deal with the changes in EMS over the last 30 years. At the heart of good education is problem-solving skills. It has never failed to amaze me that many of us spend our time in class worrying about answering questions when once we graduate, most of our professional life is spent asking *them!*

The Case of the Month column in *JEMS* has been an effort to provide challenging scenarios for the purpose of solving assessment problems. When you peel back the layers of what we really do in this field, it comes down to a patient relating to us an equation, often with many unknowns and variables. We must use this often disjointed and unreliable data to come to an extremely accurate assessment and treatment plan, often while being distracted by other uncontrollable events and people around us.

Most people would call this chaos. But for you, it is just another day at the office.

I hope that you enjoy reading and working in this collection of "equations" as much as I did writing them.

All the best,

Paul A. Werfel

Paul A. Werfel

1
PATIENT ASSESSMENT

Ignorance Is Voluntary Misfortune

"A pleasant illusion is better than a harsh reality."
—Christian N. Bovee

Why did we get into this wild west show called EMS? Was it to memorize the 14 separate steps to applying a traction splint? Definitely not. Was it to find the most "interesting" mnemonic for the cranial nerves? I doubt it. So why do we do this? What compels us to learn all the medical jargon and skills? Very simply, we love to go on calls, and we find the cases we see interesting. Sometimes tragic, sometimes difficult, sometimes more than we bargained for. Yet at the end of long shifts, actual cases are what keep us coming back for more.

My name is Paul Werfel, I'm a paramedic and, yes, what keeps me interested in EMS are the cases we are called to manage. I am also the director of the paramedic program at the State University of New York at Stony Brook, which makes me very interested in education. The two go together. One of the best ways to learn is by looking at actual cases.

Of course, the idea of discussing cases and using them in

the EMS classroom is neither new nor revolutionary, but in many places we continue to teach hard facts. For example, we try to memorize the side effects of lidocaine or remember how many pounds of pressure to place on the defibrillator paddles, when, quite honestly, what we need to be thinking about is real situations and then learning what is needed to manage those situations.

Recently, many educators and credentialing organizations have recognized that the cases are what really matter, and no matter how many hard facts you learn, it's what you do out there on the street that really counts (what a revelation). It makes sense to train as you work and work as you train. Considering cases always stimulates divergent points, which makes learning more active and long-term. The more involved we can become in the actual cases, the more interesting and educational the experiences become—not to mention fun.

The beauty of considering cases is that they always lead to the one word question, "Why?" In my opinion, "Why?" is what EMS (and most other) education is all about. Knowing why is the concept that frees us from the toils of being simple robots. We must be why-driven EMS practitioners to deal with the demands that will be made on our profession in the future.

Scenario

So let's consider a case. An elderly lady bends over to pick up her five-year-old granddaughter. The child accidentally kicks her in the abdomen. She presents to the EMS crew with "the worst stomach pain she has ever felt." The pain is in the vicinity of the umbilicus. All vital signs are stable, and the crew performs a thorough assessment. They examine her abdomen and find nothing. There is no bruising. The belly is soft with no masses. So off to the hospital they go.

Upon arrival, the physician examines the patient, and the recorded vital signs are pulse 80, BP 150/90, resp 18. The physician essentially finds the same thing as the prehospital practitioners. The woman's belly hurts, but she has a soft abdomen with no rebound, rigidity or guarding. In this scenario, the patient is then evaluated by the trauma surgeons, admitted and scheduled for a CT scan the next day. During the night, the patient suffers a cardiorespiratory arrest and is pronounced 40 minutes later. A sad story, but what is there for us to garner here?

Those of you who have taken PALS and other courses know that kids respond to the stress of trauma and illness quite differently than adults. What some of us are as yet to be cognizant of is that the elderly also respond very differently to these same stresses. What are some of these differences?

Diminished ability to raise the heart rate. This means that you may not see the tachycardia you would expect to see in the younger adult. In addition, the oldster may be taking medications that will further reduce the ability to increase heart rate in response to stress (beta/calcium channel blocking agents or digitalis).

Reduced ability to vasoconstrict. This means that we may not see the pallor and cool skin we expect to see in early or compensated shock. This and the inability to raise the heart rate basically remove two of the parameters in our assessment of shock.

Abdominal injuries in the elderly are often occult. Why is this the case? As we age, our perception of pain begins to decrease. This can be due to mental or hearing difficulties, increasing pain tolerance or the inability of the patient to precisely locate the painful area.

These, dear reader, are the keys for our understanding of this patient's demise. An autopsy finds that the patient had a ruptured intestine, profuse internal bleeding and diffuse peritonitis (fecal matter throughout her abdominal cavity) that caused her death. What would have happened if this patient had been 40 years old? She would have been in the OR much quicker. Why? Because the younger patient would probably have presented with the vaunted "boardlike abdomen" and rapid heart rate, necessitating rapid surgical exploration.

It is for these reasons and others that the elderly have nearly five times the death rate for abdominal trauma than other age groups because:

- The elderly may not respond to abdominal trauma the way we expect.
- The signs of trauma may be less obvious.
- Older patients are less tolerant of surgery to begin with. They tend to be very susceptible to post-op lung problems and infections.
- Older patients with abdominal trauma require a high degree of suspicion.

Being suspicious is at the very core of the prehospital being. Isn't that what we are here for? Our job is to see beyond the obvious and then entertain our suspicions. When we see a 50-year-old with epigastric pain, we think beyond the claim of indigestion. The same is true with trauma. Look at the mechanism of injury. If it's possible that something is injured, let us proceed as though it is. Make sure we think of horses when we hear hoofbeats, and not zebras.

Expose Yourself

"Where there is no vision, the people perish."
—*Proverbs 29:18*

Do you remember the Alfred Hitchcock film *Psycho*? No
doubt those of you who do probably felt trepidation
about showering in a motel for some time after seeing
the movie. Why was the shower scene so frightening?
Clearly it wasn't the act of murder itself because we
never saw a knife touch Janet Leigh's flesh in the movie.
And we see more graphic and violent acts every day on
network TV. I think the scene was so terrifying to the
audience because we all feel exposed standing naked in
the shower and could relate to Leigh's vulnerability.
Most people think being exposed is a bad thing, and in
many cases they are correct. Is exposure ever a beneficial
state? Let's examine this case to find out.

Scenario
You're working with your regular partner, Connie, who

just graduated from paramedic school. She's a competent medic who needs more experience to hone her skills. You decide to drive throughout this shift to give Connie more "tech" time.

As the two of you debate whose family gets more dysfunctional around the holidays, the dispatcher requests your presence at a "shooting with multiple victims, the Stapleton Housing Projects, 2453 Schaeffer Blvd., cross street of McCormick." As you weave through the evening traffic, your mind clicks off the possibilities for injuries on scene and also the assets you'll need should this be a full-fledged mass-casualty incident. The police dispatcher updates you that the call is actually for a drive-by shooting and reports that you have only one victim with minor injuries. As you roll up, the police direct you to an 18-year-old male wearing a dark hooded sweatshirt. The victim tells you he heard gunfire coming from a car and jumped off his porch head first to get flat on the sidewalk. He had his hands in front of him (like a dive into a swimming pool) and landed flat on his chest. He's complaining of left-side chest pain and states that he was not shot. He has no history and takes no medications.

The police officer suggests that the patient probably broke a rib diving for the deck. As you place the patient on oxygen, Connie gets his vitals: Pulse 100, BP 96/70, respirations 20 and shallow. Lung sounds are clear and equal on both sides. She palpates the chest though the sweatshirt and doesn't feel any crepitus.

Things look OK as you place the patient on the stretcher. Connie wants to place an IV to keep the vein open just in case of problems. You agree, and she establishes the IV line during the unhurried ride to the hospital. During transport, the patient begins complaining of some shortness of breath and feeling light-headed. Connie attributes this to the pain associated with the rib fracture. She turns up the oxygen and decides to take a look at the patient's chest. She slices the shirt up the middle and examines the patient's anterior—good, no trauma or other obvious defects. But soon the patient begins having profound difficulty breathing and is losing consciousness. Connie tells you to rush to the hospital as she ventilates and attempts to intubate the patient. The intubation attempt is unsuccessful, and the patient arrests.

On arrival at the hospital, the trauma team completely removes the patient's sweatshirt and other clothing. They notice that the patient's neck veins are distended. As they lift his arms, they find a small round hole about the size of a pencil eraser in the patient's armpit. A chest tube is placed on the side of the wound, and the tension pneumothorax is relieved.

Unfortunately, relief did not come quickly enough for the patient, as you find out during your next meeting with your medical director and supervisor. He regained pulses but remained brain dead. Due to his IV drug history, the patient was deemed unsuitable as an organ/tissue donor. He was removed from life support and died soon thereafter.

Would prehospital discovery of the bullet wound have made a difference? At the very least, its discovery would have caused the transport to be expedited—perhaps with different results. For most of us, the thought of being exposed—whether legally or otherwise—is a cause for dread. Conversely, in some situations, such as when you are evaluating a trauma patient, the failure to completely expose the patient to your critical eye is a situation that should be cause for similar apprehension.

Connie allowed herself to be led down the wrong assessment path by a patient who could not visualize or feel the existing wound. It is our job to assess each patient based on what we see and know about the incident. In my book, a patient who was shot at and reports pain and/or trauma has been hit until I can determine otherwise through a thorough assessment that includes a complete visualization—exposure—and palpation of the patient's entire body.

Watchful Eye

"The price of freedom is eternal vigilance."
—*Wendell Phillips*

When he said this, Wendell Phillips, an American reformer and anti-slave activist in the 1800s, could have been speaking about a career in EMS. Most of us agree that our training programs were anything but easy. We endured hours and hours of study, nebulous facts, endless reading assignments and weekly tests—all for relentless instructors whose demands seemed endless. In a manner of speaking, we had to keep a vigilant watch on how we did in class to avoid problems along the way.

Similarly, once finished with our training programs, we had to remember that the most effective item we bring to our patient's bedside is vigilance—the critical eye that observes and makes decisions on the patient's condition. To bring this powerful tool to bear, we need to remember that we must observe the patient. Sounds like child's play doesn't it? Let's examine this case and see.

Scenario

You're working at your part-time job for a private ambulance service that does mostly inter-facility transfers. Your partner, Vinnie "The Vin-Man" Barrano is also a part-timer, as well as a full-time EMS supervisor ("brass" as he likes to say) at a local hospital. He's the kind of medic who has four different hemostats on his utility belt.

As you ride around, Vinnie (the world's foremost authority on his own opinion) attempts to convey the merits of professional wrestling and its position as a legitimate sport. Luckily, your dispatcher breaks up the conversation and assigns you to a "psychiatric transfer going from Boyd Memorial Hospital to the Fending-Sontag Psychiatric Rehabilitation Hospital." Dispatch also informs you that the physician at Boyd has not requested that you restrain the patient. As you proceed to the assignment, you reflect on the appropriateness of the call, because at the moment you're driving with Vin-Man the wrestling maniac.

Your vehicle arrives at the transferring hospital. You and Vinnie are presented with a 30-year-old male who has been depressed lately and has harbored suicidal thoughts, according to the ED physician. The social worker and psychiatrist have seen the patient and agree that he needs treatment at the psych hospital.

The Boyd staff didn't restrain the patient and again state that he doesn't need to be restrained in your vehicle for the half-hour ride. You obtain vitals and find that the patient, Eric Parsley, is a musician with a history of emotional problems that have worsened in the past week. The patient record confirms that he doesn't take any drugs presently and has no other pertinent medical history.

As you sit in the captain's chair behind the patient, writing portions of your report, he asks if you wouldn't mind sitting him up a little. You place the stretcher at about 45°, but the patient still insists that he is uncomfortable. Grudgingly, you lift the back until the patient is sitting just about upright. Now on the interstate, you settle back into your seat, filling out the rest of the run report, while your partner tunes in the theme from *Saturday Night Fever* on the radio. As you turn to look for the mileage, your patient stands up, gets the back door open and jumps out of the vehicle. As you watch transfixed, he is struck by one vehicle, and another and another.

The outcome is predictable. The patient is dead and you and your partner are stunned beyond words. You have difficult questions to answer and lose a lot of sleep over this situation. There's more than enough blame to go around. Your employer wants to know why the patient was not restrained by the sending facility. The hospital attorney wants to know why you sat on the captain's chair and not on the crew bench watching the patient. The attorney throws salt on your wounds by asserting that you might have wrestled the patient down or warned your partner so he could pull the vehicle onto the shoulder.

There are some good lessons to learn from this case. Paying attention to your patient will keep you and your patient out of trouble. Clearly, the price of your job and good name may be eternal vigilance.

Take a Bite out of Assessment

"Diligence is the mother of good luck."
—*Benjamin Franklin,* Poor Richard's Almanac, *1735*

Do you believe in luck? What is luck, anyway? People define luck as fortune, chance, a flip of the coin, the way the cookie crumbles, the ship that finally came in, being at home when opportunity knocked and, perhaps, a failure's explanation for someone else's success. Does luck, either good or bad, play a part in our patient outcomes? Let's examine this case to find out.

Scenario—Do you know your ABCs?

You're an instructor and a paid paramedic first responder with the local volunteer fire department. You're the only one on duty at the station. After checking the contents of your ALS-equipped Suburban and the department ambulances, you settle in with your coffee and newspaper. As you enjoy the sunrise, you hear alert tones come over the radio. Dispatch announces: "Collision, heavy rescue required; Old Field Road., cross street, West Meadow Ave. Time out is 0602."

As you pull up, you see a single compact car that had hit a traffic signal on the driver's side door. You can tell the car had been traveling at a relatively high rate of speed because it is actually bent in the area of the driver's door. Neither door opens. Inside you locate two patients, both restrained and in their 60s. By this time the fire chief, an ambulance and the department's rescue company are also en route to the scene.

You find the female passenger alert and talking, but the male driver is unresponsive. An EMT bystander is leaning through a broken window and holding the man's head. He tells you that he removed the driver's false teeth to help him breathe. You get into the car through the hatchback and take over C-spine control of the driver. You see a set of false teeth at the patient's feet. The EMTs who arrived on the ambulance place an oropharyngeal airway (OPA), administer high-flow oxygen and apply a cervical collar.

While the EMTs attend to the female passenger and someone else takes over C-spine control, you assess the driver. You find an unconscious patient, breathing at a rate of 22 with good bilateral breath sounds, but some bruises from the steering wheel on his chest. His pulse is 80, blood pressure 148/80. He responds only to painful stimuli. His pelvis is unstable, and he has obvious fractures to the left upper and lower arm. In addition, his lower legs remain trapped under the mangled dashboard.

The rescue company works to free your patient as you establish an IV and monitor vital signs. After 20 minutes, they liberate your patient, and you place him on a backboard for transport to University Hospital emergency department (ED). As you place the patient in the ambulance, you reassess his airway. You remove the OPA, apply suction to clear blood in the airway and decide to intubate the patient to locate the source of the bleeding. Under direct vision of the laryngoscope, you clearly visualize both vocal cords—and, squarely between the cords, the bottom section of the patient's false teeth.

You carefully remove the lower denture with Magill forceps and place the endotracheal tube. By this time, your ambulance is pulling up to the emergency entrance at the hospital, where you release the patient to the trauma team.

Lessons learned
As you reflect on this case, you decide to add some notes to your next lecture:

Lesson 1: There are exceptions to every rule. You never heard the oft-mentioned stridor that's considered the gold standard in upper airway obstructions.

Lesson 2: Always revisit the ABCs once your patient has been immobilized and is accessible. This will prove a great shield to avoid disaster and embarrassment.

Lesson 3: Always recheck the airway for obstructions after the patient has been extricated. The oropharynx may appear clear while the patient remains trapped in the seat, but they can still have a life-threatening airway obstruction farther down the airway.

Lesson 4: When you find one denture, you'll most often find another. Always account for both dentures— upper and lower.

Throughout history, people have sought to explain the inexplicable and unexpected things that happen to people. Someone hits the lottery; another dies in a freak accident. People have used religion, superstition, actuarial tables and dreams to explain this. Although luck does have a place in EMS, we must remember that education, experience and attention to detail create their own luck.

Don't forget: The sale of good luck charms and tokens may be a healthy industry, but that rabbit's foot on your key chain didn't bring much luck to its original owner.

Mental Triage

"What a man hears, he may doubt. What he sees, he may possibly doubt. But what he does, he cannot doubt."

—*Anonymous*

As EMS practitioners, we must do some rather distasteful things in our daily routine. Asking personal questions, such as, "Is it possible that you're pregnant?" or "When was your last menstrual period, Ma'am?" never gets easy. While conducting these uncomfortable interrogations, we must often make judgments that may have a great impact on others. As a matter of fact, we make these judgments so often, we may not remember the impact they may have.

Determining death is one such judgment call. How often have you had to terminate care because your efforts were unsuccessful? How do you know a person is dead and beyond your capabilities to resuscitate them? A great fear among citizens trained in CPR or neophyte EMS providers: They won't know if a person is dead. Sometimes it isn't obvious. Mistakes can happen, as we see in this case.

Scenario

The dispatcher sends you to a "cardiac arrest at the Short Manufacturing Company, 1204 Jay Street, corner of Hellmann Blvd. Time is 1120." You and your partner make your way to the scene, wondering what awaits you. Is it a real arrest or simply someone who's experienced a syncopal episode on a hot day?

You pull in front of the factory and see folks waving you to the front door. They tell you their coworker, Bill, went into cardiac arrest, and bystanders resuscitated him. You make your way to the patient and find a 48-year-old male complaining of chest pain, lightheadedness and difficulty breathing. He denies heart trouble and says his only pertinent history is an ulcer. He denies taking any medication. He describes the pain as sharp and worsening when he breathes. He's alert and oriented x 3, and his lung sounds are clear. He denies any history of asthma and doesn't smoke.

Your partner places the patient on oxygen and applies a cardiac monitor. The patient points to exactly where it hurts—on the right side of his sternum, where the third and fourth ribs join the breastbone. The patient's ECG demonstrates sinus tachycardia with a rate of 120, and his blood pressure is 84/70.

The monitor shows no other ectopy. "Maybe he has a leaking aneurysm in his chest," you think. The explanation fits, but he's young and doesn't have a history of hypertension or anything else that would signify an aneurysm. His lung sounds are good (what you can hear of them because he's taking shallow breaths), so pneumothorax probably isn't the issue.

While your partner starts an IV, you speak to the

bystanders who performed CPR. They tell you the patient got up from his workstation, complained of being lightheaded and then passed out. They say they began CPR, and in a few seconds he woke up and complained of chest pain.

You direct your attention back to the patient and decide, along with your partner, to postpone treating his cardiac symptoms and search for the origin of his chest pain. You begin a more focused physical assessment and obtain the patient history. He claims his stomach doesn't hurt, but he still feels dizzy and his chest hurts.

As you mentally review the facts, an idea occurs to you. You put your hand on the spot where he claims his pain is the worst. You palpate an abnormal bump in the area. His pain increases as you press on it. You tell him to take the deepest breath he can take. When he does so, you feel movement in the area and the patient screams in pain. *The problem:* His sternum separated from the rib when the bystanders performed CPR.

Armed with the knowledge the patient's probably not having an MI, you ask for more of his history en route and find that he noticed his stools have looked black during the past two weeks, indicating a possible GI bleed. The transport goes without incident.

The patient subsequently receives a blood transfusion at the hospital for a bleeding ulcer and has his rib-sternal separation treated as a complication to his primary problem.

Discussion

In EMS, our job is to sort through the confusing, conflicting and often incorrect information on scene, make a decision about what's wrong with our patients and do something about it. As in the case above, when we're proficient in mental triage, we can solve just about any complex case.

Reasonable Doubt

*"I respect faith, but it is doubt
that gets you an education."*
—Wilson Mizner

An instructor once told me that experience and doubt were the dividends that he got from his mistakes. Most of us go through life doubting certain things and events. We read the newspapers and watch TV, concerned about the truth of the stories reported. We wonder if overtime pay will show up in this week's check. We wonder if we really will get the new ambulance assigned to our platoon when it's ready for service.

In EMS, we harbor doubts about our patients, partners, bosses, coworkers—even ourselves. Each time we respond to a call we perform live. We can't redo an assignment later if we make mistakes on the first try. We need a multipurpose "device" to ensure the job gets done well and to make the job safer for our patients and ourselves. Healthy doubt, an important skill for prehospital practitioners, may be the "Swiss army knife" we're looking for, as this case illustrates.

Scenario

It's a wonderful fall day: The leaves are changing colors; a cool wind kicks up. You and your partner are stopped at a nearby park watching some kids fly their kites when the dispatcher assigns you to "a male with abdominal pain at the LaMonica State Hospital, 2nd floor of the Theodore Unit. Time 0932."

Oh great—a bellyache at LaMonica. The staff members there wait until a patient has one foot in the grave and another on a banana peel before they call for EMS.

On arrival, you're escorted to the bedside of a 43-year-old male with what appears to be excruciating abdominal pain. The nurse tells you that the pain began about four hours ago and has worsened since then. The patient, who is alert and oriented x 3, tells you the pain began intermittently in his navel area and has progressed to his entire abdomen. He says the pain is constant and begs you to do something to ease it.

His vital signs are BP 130/80; pulse 90 and irregular; respirations 18 and regular. The electrocardiogram shows atrial fibrillation with a rate of 90. The patient has normal skin color. There are no other abdominal signs or symptoms. The abdomen is soft with no tenderness or masses.

The nurse at LaMonica tells you the patient received an artificial heart valve about seven months ago and has been treated for chronic atrial fibrillation for the past five years with digoxin and propranolol. The nurse also informs you that the patient's doctor has seen him and does not believe his complaints to be genuine. When the patient says he's feeling better and asks to sign a release so he can go back to bed, you're briefly tempted to leave him, especially because his vitals and history are OK. But he's hurting and that worries you and your partner.

You doubt the patient is acting out and remember that, unlike chest pain (where the problem is usually in the heart or lungs), abdominal pain involves several organs and a variety of pains and locations. You convince the patient he should be evaluated at the hospital, make him comfortable, give him oxygen and begin transport. All routine.

Days later, you learn your doubts probably saved this guy's life. Emboli obstructed his mesenteric artery and about a foot of his small intestine was necrotic. The ED physician who treated your patient tells you that abdominal pain out of proportion to the patient's appearance is the classic presentation of mesenteric infarct. He adds that this disproportion can be caused by atrial fibrillation or artificial heart valves. The mortality rate for such a patient runs 70–90% because health-care providers often don't suspect it, delaying diagnosis.

The Chinese character for crisis is a combination of two other characters—danger and opportunity. In EMS we see crises daily. For us, the danger lies in possible oversights that may affect our patients. The opportunities lie in helping our patients and keeping ourselves out of trouble. Doubts are healthy. They shield us from the risks that wait in the crises we encounter.

20 Tips to Perfect Your Assessment Skills

There are two reasons we learn patient assessment early in our EMS training programs: First, without a sound patient assessment, the skills we work so tirelessly to perfect (e.g., CPR, spinal immobilization, defibrillation, IV starts) would be worthless to us because we would never know when to use them.

Second, assessment is an art and, as such, it takes a significant portion of an EMS training program to polish our technique to the point that we don't miss any important item of patient information. This fine tuning of our assessment methodology usually continues for some time after completion of the program. We must become why-driven instead of simply concerning ourselves with manual skills. Here are 20 important assessment tips I've learned over the years and would like to pass on to you.

General patient assessment

1 We're in the information business. The most important part of patient assessment is the vectored, logical accumulation of complete patient information. Although we use some skills and procedures with regu-

larity (taking a blood pressure, starting an IV or evaluating an ECG), we perform others only rarely in the course of our practice (needle cricothyrotomy, intraosseous infusions).

The anchor of our practice is the skill we perform on every patient: assessment. It's frequently the most challenging thing we do. Why? Each patient is different. Some are excellent historians and can tell you the whys, whens and hows of their conditions. Some are afraid to admit they could be seriously ill.

Others are non-communicative or unaware of their conditions, medications or hospitalizations. Often the patient's families or caregivers don't offer much help. It has always amazed me that folks can live with loved ones for decades and not know anything about such important things as their medical conditions or the medications they take.

Take the time, make the connection with the patient and get them to talk to you.

2 There are more illnesses than protocols to treat them. Unfortunately, many EMS practitioners become protocol-driven. They feel the patient needs to fit into the nice, comforting pigeonhole of a specific protocol. The reality is that most of the disease entities we come across do not have a corresponding protocol. Most of us don't have a headache protocol or an upset stomach protocol. Although applying the one-size-fits-all approach that protocols give us may provide an anchor in a sea of uncertainty, its parochial approach is extremely limiting.

3 Diabetics, women and the elderly may have atypical MI presentations. We know diabetics frequently lose feeling in their toes and extremities. But we sometimes

forget that they lose feeling in their hearts as well. Fact is, 45% of folks older than 70 do not have chest pain as a symptom of a heart attack.

Diabetics and the elderly with heart attacks present with fatigue, shortness of breath, neck, back or arm pain, toothache, jaw pain or abdominal pain—either singly or in combination. Thirty percent of elderly patients with MI (and even more diabetics with MI) have silent events that exhibit no symptoms.

Usually, women don't get ischemic heart disease until menopause. Once menopausal, they suffer heart attacks as often as men and die more often. Remember that female patients suffering a cardiac event frequently present with abdominal pain—not chest pain.

4 Assessing patients who've consumed alcohol or drugs is difficult. Does your patient have an altered level of consciousness because they are intoxicated or under the influence of drugs? Or is it because they are bleeding in their brain? Patients on drugs or alcohol are not forthcoming or accurate about their medical histories. Getting reliable and accurate information from such patients may be among your greatest assessment challenges. Use bystanders, friends and family members to help fill in the blanks.

Medical patients
5 All that wheezes is not asthma. We get so used to hearing asthmatics wheeze that we often forget that patients with other serious problems exhibit wheezing. Conditions like anaphylaxis, pneumonia and pulmonary embolus may cause a patient to wheeze. Early pulmonary edema and congestive heart failure commonly present with wheezing—not the expected crackles or

rales. That's why it's called cardiac asthma.

6 Women with abdominal pain need to go to the hospital for evaluation. Women of childbearing age can experience an ectopic pregnancy, something you don't want to assess as simple abdominal pain. The rate of occurrence is approximately one in 200 pregnancies. Ectopic pregnancy is the leading cause of first trimester fetal death in the United States and causes more than 11% of all maternal deaths in this country. This condition is the great imitator. Symptoms vary: abdominal pain, with or without vaginal bleeding or spotting, nausea and vomiting.

The patient's menstrual history is often inconclusive, with the absence of menses varying as well. Leaving these patients to visit their own physician the next day will earn you poor style points if they bleed to death. Use all your powers of persuasion to get them to go to the hospital.

7 People with dizzy spells often have serious arrhythmias, GI bleeds or neurologic emergencies. Frequently, the first symptom of a serious arrhythmia, stroke or internal bleeding from an ulcer is dizziness or syncope. Such patients are lightheaded when they stand and may eventually fall. Hence the fact that many of these alarms come in as a fall. Be suspicious.

8 An aspirin a day can keep the cardiologist away, but can get you to the gastroenterologist quicker. Is aspirin a great drug for patients with suspected MIs or as a preventive measure to reduce the risk of a heart attack? Sure. Are there problems with taking it every day? Yes again. Since physicians began telling their patients to

take an aspirin each day, many people have felt that they can benefit from this wonder drug. *The downside:* Prolonged aspirin intake can cause ulcers and other bleeding conditions in the gastrointestinal tract. When confronted with a patient suffering from abdominal pain, always ask about their aspirin intake.

Trauma patients

9 Hypotension is a late sign of shock. In most patients, the first signs of shock are cool, clammy, pale skin and a rapid pulse. During the early stages of blood loss, the patient's blood pressure may actually rise slightly. Once the patient loses 30% of their blood volume, decompensated shock occurs and the patient's BP drops.

10 Adults cannot become hypotensive due exclusively to closed head trauma. Adults with closed head trauma cannot have a low blood pressure and elevated pulse rate due to blood loss in the head. There is simply not enough space to put the requisite amount of blood to throw your patient into shock.

In adult patients with closed head trauma and unstable vital signs, look for other injuries and bleeding in the usual suspect areas: the chest, abdomen, pelvis and femurs. Conversely, due to their proportionately larger heads, pediatric patients can have a low BP and rapid heart rate due to blood loss in the head.

11 Short boards and traction splints work well for stable trauma victims—not for unstable ones. Although these immobilization devices are great for stable patients with C-spine injuries or femur fractures, unstable patients with C-spine injuries must be quickly extricated and rapidly transported to a trauma center.

Likewise, an unstable patient with a femur fracture can be best managed by tying their legs together, placing them on a longboard and moving them to the trauma center. It does our patients no good to arrive at a trauma center perfectly packaged, but in cardiac arrest.

12 The multiple-trauma patient with head trauma and shock needs to be treated like any other multi-trauma victim. In our zeal not to worsen a patient's intracranial pressure, we often undertreat their blood-loss problem. This leads to hypoperfusion, which creates more problems for the injured brain. The brain needs blood flow and oxygen to recover from injuries (including elevated intracranial pressure). In addition, irreversible shock will do your patient in much faster than intracranial pressure. Reduce heat loss, position your patient properly and maintain perfusion to their brain.

Geriatric patients

13 Geriatric patients may never exhibit tachycardia, pallor or hypotension from blood loss. Note the normal changes that occur in the cardiovascular system as a result of aging. Elderly patients have a profound reduction in their ability to raise their heart rates. Why? As we age, we have a diminished response to the hormones in our body that increase the heart rate and constrict our blood vessels. The specialized tissues in our hearts that carry electrical impulses tend not to conduct the electric signals as fast as we age. Therefore, our cardiac output drops by 30% between ages 30 and 80.

Why is this important? If the elderly cannot raise their heart rates, what happens when they are injured and become hypovolemic? Will they present with tachycardia or pallor? Probably not. This does not even take into account that many elderly people take medications that further reduce their heart rate.

This results in the loss of one of shock's early warning signs. When we add to this the fact that many older people have hypertension, we may see blood pressures in the 112/70 range that we would not classify as hypotension in a young person, but is seriously low for a person who's normal BP is 160/90.

14 Differentiate acute problems from chronic ones. Elderly patients tend to have several illnesses simultaneously. It is not unusual for a patient to have hypertension coexisting with heart disease, diabetes, COPD and a touch of pneumonia. When this patient complains of difficulty breathing, it requires Solomon-like wisdom to search out the cause of the problem.

Are the crackles and rales that we hear when listening to the patient's chest due to pulmonary edema, or have they been present for months because the patient is confined to bed? Is the patient's skin turgor poor because of dehydration, or is it normal skin aging? These chronic conditions conspire to make the assessment perplexing.

Are you witnessing a new problem or a chronic one? If a caregiver is present, the big payoff question is, "Is this the way they usually look?"

15 The elderly can have MIs and catastrophic abdominal problems with little or no pain. *Remember:* As we age, our response to pain diminishes. This makes heart and abdominal problems difficult to detect because we key in on the patient's complaint of chest or abdominal pain. Thus, you (and the patient) may underestimate the severity of the problem. Remain particularly suspicious of elderly patients who complain about

fatigue, back and neck pain and lightheadedness.

16 Medications may disclose the patient history more reliably than the patient can. We need to know what medicines a patient takes for a simple reason: The medication is written history, not subject to much interpretation. Has a patient ever said they have no heart history, only to tell you that they take nitroglycerin, furosemide, digoxin and propranolol? Do you believe the patient or the medications you find?

Pediatric patients

17 Children are not adults who have been left in the dryer too long. We do not assess children in the same manner that we assess adults because their means of coding and exiting this world differ. When was the last time you saw a three-year-old heart attack patient? Children die from respiratory failure and shock. The next tips will key you into the assessment of these small citizens.

18 Crying, screaming children are usually stable. Here are some easy questions: Is a child screaming like a motor siren moving good air? Is their color good? As my dear friend from North Dakota says, "You betcha." Children who scream at the top of their lungs are stable for now. The children we most need to concern ourselves with are the quiet ones.

19 Blood pressure is an unreliable sign of pediatric shock. Children have healthy hearts and blood vessels. They can compensate for blood loss extremely well for short periods of time. They may maintain what you consider a good BP until 50% of blood loss occurs. This

means that you cannot depend on BP to tell you about a child's cardiovascular status. By the time the blood pressure drops, your patient is circling the eternal drain.

Look for early signs of shock in kids, such as altered level of consciousness, color, a drop in extremity temperature, the presence or absence of distal pulses and poor capillary refill (a dependable sign in kids, but not in adults) to give you the heads-up on pediatric shock

20 Lethargy and minimal response to painful stimuli in children is ominous. Normal children are active and loud most of the time. My wife and I can attest to that. I think about the noise that my six-year-old makes when she skins her knee in a fall off her bicycle or how my nine-year-old reacts to an ear infection. Children are exquisitely responsive to painful stimuli. The absence of that expected response to pain in medical or trauma situations is a foreboding and ominous finding in children.

Conclusion
File these assessment tips in your memory so you'll be able to recall them as you assess your next patient. Remember that no two patients are alike, and protocols do not fit every patient. A thorough assessment will usually lead you down the correct path to the patient's problem and subsequent treatment.

2
TRAUMA EMERGENCIES

Walking the Tightrope

How many times in a career do you collar and backboard patients? A hundred? A thousand? Is there a purpose to this or is this just one of those rules that play in our minds and haunt us? I keep hearing past instructors pontificate about head and neck trauma, how the two are interrelated and how we live for mechanism of injury. You know, they're right. Mechanism is what we live for; it's what we do.

Mechanism is not only something to think about in trauma—it's a great thing to consider in all medical patients. The only difference is that we call it the chief complaint and history of present illness. For example, when a patient presents with retrosternal chest pain, what's the first thing you think of? Pulled muscle in the chest, costochondral cartilage inflammation? I don't think so. You think of heart attack. Is this because you can see ECG changes? No, you know ECG changes may not make an appearance for several hours if it's a heart attack. The same is true for various cardioenzyme levels

(CPK-MB, troponin, myoglobin, etc.). We think heart attack because it's one of the conditions that we don't want to miss.

Most of us are pretty comfortable with the mechanism concept, but now the people who do our research, such as emergency physicians, are thinking about changing the rules. They want to know if we need to board and collar every patient who emerges from an MVC. You know the routine: you truss up one of these folks who has no complaints and no sign of headache with a collar that fits well and the best backboard. Then the patient goes to the hospital and waits an hour on a stretcher. A nurse or doctor looks in on them and asks, "What hurts?" Their surprise answer, "My back."

Some places have already instituted protocols to limit the number of patients who must be boarded. Do you think this is a good idea? Either way, you'll find this case interesting.

Scenario
Your vehicle is dispatched to a report of a workman injured at a construction site. Armed with a backboard and a selection of collars, you and your partner proceed to the scene. The foreman directs you to an area where concrete foundations are being poured. When you get there, a workman in his 40s complains of an abrasion on his ear and a slight headache.

When you ask him how this rather unimpressive injury occurred, he tells you he tripped and fell 25 feet to a concrete floor. He denies neck pain or tenderness or loss of consciousness. He is alert and oriented x 3.

At this point, the patient turns around and points to the spot he fell from. His coworkers agree; the guy did a swan dive from about 25 feet. You and your partner are unruffled about the actual injury, but think the mechanism is as impressive as hell. The two of you resort to that often practiced, but seldom used "Standing Takedown."

You perform this skill perfectly, getting the patient on the board with essentially no movement to his neck or back. The state practical exam board would be proud. The rest of his physical examination is unremarkable: pulse 96; respiration 14; BP 134/88; PERRLA. He has no medical history, hospitalizations or medications.

You transport the patient to the trauma center. On arrival, you present the patient as a rule-out C-spine injury and go back into service. After a cappuccino, the two of you discuss how unimpressed you were with the actual injury and only boarded this guy because the mechanism looked good. You believe the possibility of the patient having a head or C-spine injury as remote, at best.

However, your partner gets on his nightly soapbox about how HMOs interfere with prehospital care by frowning on boarding and collaring of certain patients because it mandates X-rays and drives up health-care costs. You're on the verge of nulling him out, when the dispatcher sends you on another assignment.

When you arrive at the hospital with your next patient, you ask about the workman you brought in earlier. The nurse tells you the patient had unstable fractures of C-1 and C-2. You inform your partner of this turn of events and you both agree it was a good idea you immobilized him. The mechanism helped preserve your patient's health.

What's really amazing: This kind of care happens every day. We go out there and walk the tightrope. And like the tightrope walker, the terrible mistakes we make are the most subtle: a slip here, a hesitation there. But a misstep can devastate your patient. Mechanisms are in place for a reason.

Realistic Expectations

How many times do you hear the word *burnout* nowadays? I remember first hearing it two decades ago, when I started in EMS. At that time, it was not fashionable to be burned out. It also seems that it took longer to reach the burnout stage than it does now. These days, folks whose ink has not yet dried on their certification complain that they are toasty!

What causes this? Is today's level of EMS stress so intense it chars even our new practitioners like well-placed lightning strikes? Are the patients any different? Are the bosses worse? What's changed?

My opinion is that many of those who get into EMS do so for the wrong reasons. The most notable is that well-worn cliché: "I want to save lives." The problem is, of course, that all too often we don't save lives. But we can do many other worthwhile things for our patients—like caring enough to talk to them, as the following case demonstrates.

Scenario

Not long ago, the 17-year-old daughter of a friend was driving to her job as a lifeguard at a local water park. Three or four cars ahead of her, she saw a motorcyclist get hit by a car that had been traveling at high speed through an intersection. This young lady stopped her car to help, even though her training is limited to CPR.

She found a conscious 23-year-old with a massive evisceration and other critical injuries. She understood that there was not much she could do for this victim, but she held his hand and spoke to him. She said later she did this "so he would know he was not alone when he died." At about that time, two physicians stopped on the scene, took one look at this victim, saw the extent of the carnage and basically turned around and walked away, saying that nothing could be done. As the ambulance arrived, the victim suffered cardio-respiratory arrest. The crew began CPR and transported the victim to the trauma center, where the young man died. Several days later, my friend's daughter went to the funeral of this young man, met his parents and afterward felt much better about the entire situation. This case speaks volumes about this young lady, and about us and how we deal with the terrible things we see.

What would we "dinosaurs" have done in the same situation? We are relatively comfortable and confident when we deal with the horrors of our profession in familiar surroundings and with adequate equipment. But what can we do for our patients when their injuries are so severe that they defy the depth of our skills and the capabilities of our equipment? I propose the revival of the lost art of communicating.

Communication can be a wonderful thing. Up to now, EMS communications courses have included things like kilohertz, VHF and multiplex-duplex. But what about therapeutic communication? Talking to our patients is a great start; it is usually the easiest route for getting the information we need to administer the proper care. In addition, talking to people provides us with a way to establish rapport with patients, perhaps calming fears and, if nothing else, demonstrating to patients that they are not alone and that we care.

Why is burnout so prevalent among folks with little EMS experience? In my opinion, the problem can be blamed at least in part on television. Young people watch programs about EMS that depict the equivalent of a career's worth of high-profile assignments in a half hour. And, of course, all the patients survive. The mundane nature of our jobs and the value of communicating with all patients are definitely not stressed in these shows. Impressionable people watch and decide that they want to be a part of the excitement and the hero worship exhibited by the grateful relatives seen in these shows.

These people start EMS work and quickly realize that to get on the front page of the newspaper with a high-profile assignment, they have to labor on perhaps hundreds of routine cases. They soon discover that the cardiac arrest save rate in their area is not comparable to the one that was demonstrated on Rescue 9-1-1. Disappointment sets in.

This reminds me of the time my wife and I, as new homeowners, watched *This Old House* and *Hometime* and expected to remove all the wallpaper on the second floor and to refinish the kitchen cabinets—all on one Saturday afternoon. After all, it only took a half hour on TV! Fatigue rapidly replaced our initial excitement.

This is the same reaction we see in new EMS providers, and it is made worse by poor communication skills. These people quickly tire and quit. How do we combat this? We should help them and ourselves learn to be honest about our career expectations. If you don't like dealing with people, this is the wrong occupation for you.

I would like to see more practitioners in the field who act like the caring people that I know they can be, rather than those who seem to take their cues from the cutout characters on television. It's up to us, though, to choose: a caring communicator like my friend's daughter or someone interested only in unrealistic, largely silent drama.

Dynamics of Learning

"Everyone complains of his memory, and no one complains of his judgment."—La Rochefoucauld, Maxims

How do we acquire the much sought-after skill known as clinical judgment? Didn't we learn all we needed to know about prehospital medicine in our EMT or paramedic classes? 'Fraid not grasshopper! The dirty little secret is that when you graduate from EMT or paramedic class, the learning isn't over; it's just beginning.

This may be a news flash for some of you, but those written and practical exams you stressed over ensured only your minimum competency—not expertise. Surprised? Well, did your high school or college classes give you all the tools to you need to succeed? Did they offer a course to prepare you for job interviews, multi-tasking, balancing your checkbook or preparing for an IRS audit?

If these subjects were not formally taught in your classroom or ivy covered building, then how did you learn them? Experience. For some, experience means hitting the ground running and never having difficulty in a situation. Yet, as this case illustrates, for most of us experience is an eclectic combination of doing some things well and making occasional mistakes.

Scenario
Your ambulance is dispatched to a motorcyclist down. On arrival, you find an unconscious 35-year-old male. According to witnesses, he was thrown about 75 feet from where his motorcycle landed. Unfortunately, the state in which you work does not require motorcycle riders to wear helmets. You maintain in-line immobilization while your partner performs the initial assessment. Lacerations on the patient's face and the back of his head bleed profusely. While you control the bleeding, your partner takes the patient's vital signs and records them as BP 88/60, heart rate 122 and respirations of 30. Your partner notices that the respirations vary in depth. You and your partner assume that the patient has a dramatic elevation in intracranial pressure and must be transported rapidly without fluid resuscitation. At that point, assessment stops. You both also agree that you should intubate and hyperventilate the patient at a rate of 20 to 30 breaths per minute. You reason that hyperventilating will blow off the carbon dioxide and cause vasoconstriction of the blood vessels in his brain, resulting in lowered intracranial pressure. You do this and transport the patient to the trauma center.

By the time the patient arrives at the hospital, his vital signs bottom out and the ED staff initiates CPR. The surgeon listens to your presentation while the staff exposes your patient. They find a large area of ecchymosis on the left side of the patient's chest, and breath sounds are absent on the left side. The surgical team places a 14-gauge needle into the man's chest and you hear a rush of air. The patient remains in cardiac arrest and is pronounced dead 30 minutes later.

Lessons learned
We can learn several lessons from this unfortunate case. First, this guy certainly had the mechanism for chest injuries in addition to head injuries. Getting thrown 75 feet down the road simply can't help the bellows mechanism that we depend on to transport life-sustaining oxygen to our cells. The stabilization and assessment process began routinely enough. In-line immobilization was performed; the initial assessment was started; and vital signs were taken. Then the crew saw the patient's abnormal breathing patterns and stopped the assessment.

Had the crew continued, they would have found the chest injury, which ultimately became a tension pneumothorax. This is a treatable condition in many EMS systems (as it was in this case). The bigger problem here was a lack of basic information about science. When a patient has closed head trauma and is in shock, treat them like any other patient in shock. An adult cannot sequester enough blood in the head to cause shock. If you have a patient who presents with closed head trauma and shock, you must look exhaustively for other trauma or areas where hemorrhage could occur. The usual suspects include chest, abdomen, retroperitoneal space, pelvis and femurs.

Many systems have incorporated this caveat into their head trauma protocols. However, there has never been a protocol drafted that can replace the experience-forged clinical judgment of a good EMT or paramedic.

Hurry up to Slow Down

"Act as if it were impossible to fail."—*Dorothea Broude*

How many times in the course of a day do you hear the word caution? Many of us recite it regularly as a mantra: caution in administering morphine, caution in moving and splinting fractures, caution signs while driving and caution recommended by police as we approach a fight scene. It never ends.

Whether backboarding people who have fallen or taking a patient to the trauma center because they fit into the "trauma center" guidelines, caution is the backbone of EMS.

However, the concern remains that the cautions we are constantly exposed to will become as familiar as the yellow traffic lights, which flash between the red and the green. The yellow signal once indicated that a driver should proceed with caution. Today it seems to indicate to some in our high-speed society that they should speed up to avoid stopping at the light. *The danger here:* occasionally people get broadsided while rushing through an intersection.

Do we have the potential to broadside our patients by dashing through a caution signal? Let's examine this case to find out.

Scenario

At a rescue squad barbecue held at a member's home, you talk shop and enjoy yourself. The mercury hovers at 90° F. You notice a fellow crew member (the one scheduled to start his paramedic course in two days) do a perfect dive into the swimming pool. The guy swims the length of the pool underwater, but instead of surfacing, he swims directly into the end wall of the pool, striking the top of his head.

As he exits the water he has a funny look on his face. You ask if he feels OK. He tells you he bumped his head in the pool, has a twinge of neck pain and a little dizziness, but it's nothing to worry about. The rest of the guests aren't concerned by his story. You don't feel the injury is that impressive either. The patient remains alert and oriented, can move all his extremities and feels your touch.

Still, the guy just doesn't look right. You decide to stop at the red light of patient care and perform a complete assessment and precautionary treatment instead of zipping through the yellow caution light and taking unnecessary risks. You immobilize his neck. He doesn't argue. Because you don't have equipment, several members retrieve an ambulance. When they return, you place a cervical collar on the patient and perform a standing immobilization, lowering the patient and backboard as a unit onto the stretcher. With straps placed and the patient's head secured, you transport him to the hospital.

His vital signs remain within normal limits—an uneventful trip. You hope for a minor injury with no lasting damage. You now realize how hollow these words must sound to the other patients whom you have reassured because they certainly sound hollow to you right now as you fear the worst.

At the ED, the C-spine X-ray shows an unstable fracture of the fourth cervical vertebra. He will need an operation—perhaps several—as well as a long period of rehabilitation to recover. He won't attend paramedic class this year, but doctors remain optimistic about his chances for recovery.

Fortunately, this patient will recover from his injury. Several surgeries, uncomfortable rehab and raw determination will allow him to return to the rescue squad and finish the paramedic class almost two years after the injury.

Could this case have gone another way? Sure! It doesn't take much to change the scenario. If you change almost anything in this case, at best this guy can look forward to moving a wheelchair around the squad building and a lifetime of dependence. Many people say that every action, everything you do results in a positive or negative effect. In EMS, this is certainly the case.

And it's also true that a decision not to do something can have a big impact. In EMS, the things you choose not to do often have the strongest impact and the most negative results on patients.

Respect and treat the mechanism of injury. Walking a neck injury or chest pain patient to your unit, smelling alcohol and assuming it caused the syncope or encouraging a sign-off from a parent because their child landed on his feet after a two-story fall will get you—and your patient—broadsided at the intersection.

Chronic On-the-Job Fatigue

"Making predictions can be tricky, especially about the future."
—*Anonymous*

What happens when fatigue gets the best of us? Some of us think clearly and rationally, others get frustrated and angry, and some become quiet and withdrawn. Often, our reactions depend on our personality type.

Whether caused by working double shifts or the pressures of life, each of us lives with some level of fatigue. Although I know many type-A personalities who will freely admit they work their best under pressure, I have never met anyone who preferred to work while exhausted. Weariness saps our ability to perform tasks at optimal levels and creates crises out of minor annoyances. That said, how does fatigue affect our patient care? Let's inspect this case to find out.

Scenario

You and your partner are finishing a 24-hour shift on Halloween. The day has included a melange of collisions, fights (a block party that degenerated into a near riot, leaving two people stabbed and another shot) and other mayhem. As the two of you discuss the advantages of having the government declare Halloween null and void, the dispatcher requests your presence at an apartment building in the far end of your district for a 24-year-old male, injuries from an earlier motor vehicle accident.

Outstanding! A guy who could have gone to the hospital hours ago decides to wait until minutes before your shift change to call. On the way across town, you review the injuries from prior MVA assignments you have responded to over the years. You conclude that had the collision caused anything other than "insurance-itis," the patient would have gone to the hospital immediately after the accident happened.

On scene, you find a 24-year-old male sitting on a chair in his apartment. He tells you that he was in an auto accident five hours ago. He felt fine afterward, so he had a friend pick him up at the scene and take him home. Subsequently, he drank a couple beers and watched TV until his shoulders, arms and neck began to hurt. Now, he says the pain is really bad and he wants to go to the hospital.

This patient has no pertinent medical history and takes no medication. While your partner conducts the patient interview, you obtain the vital signs: BP 138/76; pulse 90; respirations 18. You palpate the patient's neck and shoulders and feel no deformities. He denies any loss of consciousness. You tell him to get his jacket and walk with you to the ambulance. You escort him to the crew bench where you seat him upright and secure his seatbelt. You start to fill out the run report as the white-and-orange taxi ride to the hospital begins.

As your partner drives, he makes a shallow turn and bumps the curb. This jolts you and the patient. As you start writing again, the patient says he feels nauseated and some numbness in his arms and legs. He looks flushed and feels warm. You get him on the stretcher and take his BP again: 88/60. You don't have much time to consider this turn of events as the patient begins to vomit. You quickly turn his head to the side and tend to the airway as your partner pulls up at the ED, where staff members take the patient inside.

You begin presenting to the physician in charge. As you speak, she abruptly turns and immediately places sandbags on either side of the patient's head and a cervical collar around his neck. She tells him not to move his neck or head. You begin to panic as she orders X-rays that quickly confirm an unstable cervical fracture with spinal cord involvement, which you now realize caused the patient's hypotension, numbness and flushing—all hallmarks of neurogenic shock. "My God, what did I do?" you ask yourself.

Perhaps you should think about what you didn't do. Are we all susceptible to this? I think so. In this case and others like it, we see the cumulative effects of stress, fatigue and overload in the way we perform the job. We need to teach folks what to expect with respect to changes in their thoughts and ideals after exposure to today's high-volume EMS environment. Unfortunately, many of us have grown more cynical than when we got into this business; we need to guard against the effects of that cynicism. Whether or not you think EMS providers suffer the effects of fatigue, one thing remains clear: Your patients certainly can.

Time Passages

"*Art is long, and time is fleeting.*"
—*Henry Wadsworth Longfellow, 1839*

Have you ever wished that the day had 36 hours instead of 24? Do you long for the days when life wasn't controlled by an omnipresent calendar—electronic or otherwise? An EMS career has more than its share of time limits and parameters: Credentials have expiration dates; skills change over time; and patient-care techniques have time limits (e.g., it takes 30 seconds to insert an endotracheal tube). We have also placed time limits on our patients' well-being—the most notable among them the "golden hour." These 60, ephemeral minutes can make the difference between life and death. Let's examine this case to better understand the value of that precious time.

Scenario
An ambulance is dispatched to a pedestrian struck by a

car on Elizabeth Street and Karen Blvd.—a local intersection where traffic moves like it's an interstate. On arrival, the crew finds an unconscious 30-year-old male with a large laceration on his forehead. The crew opens the patient's airway, stabilizes the cervical spine and administers high-flow oxygen via face mask.

On examination, the crew finds the patient's chest and abdomen bruised on the left side, an unstable pelvis and road rash on his extremities. The patient's vital signs: BP 122/70, pulse 96 and respirations 24. He seems pale. At this point, the crew chief calls for the newly established police helicopter to evacuate the patient to a trauma center 35 miles away (even though the receiving hospital they normally transport patients to is just a seven-minute ambulance ride). The police dispatcher informs the ambulance that the helicopter's estimated time of arrival is 35 minutes.

The crew stops the patient's external bleeding, starts two, large-bore saline IV lines and moves the man onto a backboard and into the ambulance. Someone asks the crew chief if he wants the patient to go to the local community hospital or wait for the helicopter. The chief insists that the patient has been stabilized and is a trauma center candidate. So the crew waits for the chopper—still another 20 minutes out.

As you wait in the back of the truck, you repeat the patient's vital signs, BP 108/70, pulse 118 and respirations shallow at 28. He remains unresponsive. It seems an eternity before you hear the chopper approach (total response: 25 minutes). The patient is moved to the helicopter—still unconscious, cyanotic and breathing agonally.

The patient expires in the helicopter and cannot be resuscitated. It turns out that he is the son of a prominent local congressman—a grieving father who promises an investigation into why the helicopter took so long to arrive on scene. Days pass, and speculation abounds regarding the chopper's supposedly extended response time. The pilot and crew answer endless questions.

Certainly, helicopter crew members were concerned that a patient with multiple injuries remained on scene for an extended period while only minutes away an ED was available where he could have been stabilized. In all, reputations were damaged and careers floundered as the usual suspects were rounded up.

Timeless lessons
Multi-trauma victims cannot be stabilized in the prehospital venue: They must be stabilized in EDs and operating rooms. Some patients must be transported to a hospital without delay, which is why ambulances have wheels and large engines. Other patients need trauma centers. If a delay ensues, the patient may be best served if taken to the nearest hospital. Arrangements for a specialty referral can be made later—once the patient is stable.

Our EMS maxims and parameters serve to remind us that time passes, and our patient's stay with us is fleeting. Make the most of it.

Avoid Preconceived Notions

"Everyone believes very easily whatever
he fears or desires."
—Jean De La Fontaine, Fables

Have you ever wanted something to happen in a certain way? At one time or another, all of us have wished that things would work out the way that would best suit us at the time. How about getting into a paramedic class? Will the supervisor's job come your way, or will you stay in your present position?

We try to construct our environment to facilitate attaining these wants and desires. We take classes to better ourselves and further our chances of advancement; this is a positive motivational response. However, in EMS, basing your assessment on the word of others without physically seeing the patient is fraught with danger. Let's examine this case to find out why believing isn't the same as seeing.

Scenario

You're working with R.J., a long-time paramedic. R.J. was an instructor at Downtown Hospital in the early 1980s and an EMS supervisor at Uptown Hospital for several years. He now works as a part-time paramedic for two city hospitals and spends hours telling you why he should be the city EMS consultant. Tuning him out, you look outside your station. The snow is really coming down—four inches in the past four hours. Only three hours to go on your shift. What you wouldn't give to stay in the barn until tour change.

The dispatcher announces, "Medic 43 Victor, respond to a man on the tracks under a train, Christian Ave. and Romano Blvd. Time is 2103." Great! On a miserable night like tonight, some nut had to jump in front of a train—and on the El, yet. (Part of your city's mass transit system is a light rail system called the subway. A portion elevated above the city streets is known as the El.)

These man-under assignments never turn out well. Patients are either hacked into confetti or are space cases—trapped in the six-inch space between the platform and the train. Because you'd rather not be outside in the bad weather for long, you hope that it's the former. The snow continues to pile up.

The police radio crackles to life as units begin to arrive. You almost wish they would say the guy is beyond help and cancel the call. Anything to get out of this weather. You arrive on scene, step out of the truck and see blood on the snow below the tracks. From above, the cops yell that the guy is dead. You know you should walk up and make sure, but with the weather this bad, you decide to take the cancellation and head back to your hospital station. You don't envy the guys from the morgue who will have to remove the body

Thirty minutes later, you and your partner are talking to the ED staff about the man under the train. As you tell the story, a call for a trauma code blares through the loudspeaker. The morgue wagon reports they're coming to the ED with a male who had both legs amputated by a train—your assignment.

Apparently the "dead" guy wasn't really dead. You've done this long enough to know the notifications that you'll now have to make and the incident reports to pen. You keep saying to yourself, "I should have checked. I should have checked."

Know yourself

In EMS, we all make mistakes. We're human, and it happens. In the unpredictable world of EMS, I find it amazing that we don't make more of them. But we must avoid making mistakes of legendary proportions. Be aware of your own biases. Past performance usually suggests future expectation when dealing with stocks or mutual funds, but transferring this principle to patient care is perilous.

If you've had three minor belly pain assignments in a single shift, is it prudent to assume the fourth is minor, as well? You could be mentally downgrading an ectopic pregnancy patient before you arrive on scene. Abdominal pain, with or without vaginal bleeding, is symptomatic of an ectopic pregnancy for a female patient of child-bearing age. Unlike a minor belly ache, ectopic pregnancy is the leading cause of first trimester fetal death and causes greater than 11% of all maternal deaths in this country.

Fitting a patient into your predetermined expectations makes you jaded and puts you in a position to miss things. Would the police in the above situation have taken your word about the status of a drunken driver? Would they take your word that an alleged assailant did not have a gun on him? We know the answer to those questions.

Don't accept other people's opinions about a patient for whom you're responsible. Trust yourself, your partner and few others in matters of import to your patients.

Memory Lapse

There's a classic story of a man who had gone to the circus as a child and returned many years later. As the man watched the circus, one of the elephants picked him up with its trunk and gently deposited him in the best seat in the tent. The man turned to his neighbor and proudly proclaimed, "The elephant remembered me from when I was here years ago. I fed him peanuts." Just then, the elephant came back, lifted his trunk, pointed it straight at the man and blew a stream of water in his face. "I forgot. I gave the nuts to him in the bag," the man said.

We would all agree that a good memory benefits EMS providers and their patients. In this business, we hope the things we forget are small and of little consequence—like forgetting to put a pillowcase on the stretcher pillow before the next call. When we forget important things that relate directly to patient care or safety issues, we can expect to hear about them for years to come. Want an example? Examine this case.

Scenario

You're working the last two hours of a 12-hour shift. Your partner today, Henry Hansel, used to be paramedic director of the hospital you work for. After several years of antagonizing his bosses, Hansel was dismissed from his supervisory position, but was allowed to continue working as a street paramedic.

The dispatcher calls you for a "child, possible amputation, 133-A Camille Boulevard, corner of Dexter Drive." As you drive toward the assignment, you hope the injury turns out to be a scrape that's being "up-triaged." You also ponder where to transport the patient. The nearest trauma center is 20 minutes away by ground transport, and the nearest replant site is an hour by air. Listening to the police radio, you hear the cops calling for a medical helicopter.

On arrival, you find a chaotic scene: A 12-year-old male has had his left arm severed by a band saw just below the elbow. The cops tell you that the child began playing with the saw in the garage when his father went inside to answer the phone.

As you control the bleeding with pressure, your adrenaline is flowing. You try to settle down and fight the rush because you know that mistakes are made under such conditions. Your patient exam reveals no other injuries, and the child's vital signs remain stable. Hansel administers oxygen, and you move both the patient and severed arm into your unit. Medical control has cleared the patient for air transport to the region's replant center because he's in otherwise stable condition. Hansel starts an IV as you drive to the landing zone.

You can tell that Hansel is wired. He always gets like this before a flight. Helicopters bring out the kid in many responders, but Hansel's a real rotor groupie. You pull up at the landing zone. The Bell 412 flares and touches down. Hansel and the BLS crew dispatched to assist at the landing zone load the kid into the chopper and lift off for the hour flight to the replant center.

As you drive back to the station to restock and clean the vehicle, you reflect on the injury and the impact it may make on the patient's life. Painful surgery, rehab, a loss of some function (if he's lucky) or a prosthesis.

You pull up to the station, open the side door to the patient compartment and feel a sudden wave of nausea. The patient's arm, wrapped in its moist dressing, lies in the door well. In his bluster, Hansel forgot to transfer it to the helicopter with the patient for the trip to the replant center. You get cold sweats and wonder if the child's life—or yours—will ever be the same.

Fortunately, the ending is happy for the patient. The helicopter flew back to retrieve the extremity and transported it to the replant center, where surgeons successfully reattached it.

It could happen to you
Although not as noteworthy as this, similar events happen everywhere: Units respond to calls without necessary equipment—stretcher, drug kits or other vital gear—on board. Sometimes crews leave equipment behind at the hospital in their haste to answer another call. Other times, they leave it at the station after becoming preoccupied in a conversation while checking their unit.

All of us know when our adrenaline overtakes our reactions. That's when you should take a deep breath and realize that you may be allowing events to control your responses. Remember what you must do for your patients, and do it.

Many of you accomplish this by getting the patient

in the ambulance and off a precarious scene quickly and treating them in a calmer environment. Your situational awareness can act as a safety check in the face of memory lapses. If you do have a memory lapse, you hope your patients won't suffer for your oversight, and you'll only hear a minimum of snickering in the locker room. In the worst case, your patient will suffer, and you'll hear about it at a deposition and in a courtroom and relive your oversight many times over.

If Patients Came with Instructions

"Vision is the art of seeing things invisible."
—*Jonathan Swift,* Thoughts on Various Subjects

It seems that nowadays everything comes with a safety warning or a disclaimer. We can understand why guns come equipped with trigger safeties. Ladders sold at home improvement stores have placards warning of the perils of misuse. Even coffee cups come with the warning that "contents are hot" to ostensibly avoid litigation should someone dump said contents on their lap. Wouldn't it be nice if our critical patients came with similar warnings and disclaimers to raise our caution level? This case features a patient who clearly could have used one.

Scenario
You've been dispatched to "a motor vehicle collision on O'Connor Street between Daniel Place and Golemme Boulevard. Time out: 1501." Dispatch sends a BLS unit to assist.

On arrival, you find a car has hit a utility pole and

observe at least one victim on the roadway. No electrical hazards appear present, so you approach the vehicle. A police officer alerts you to the presence of two patients, one of whom was ejected and is now "likely"—police parlance for likely to die. She also tells you the patients weren't wearing seatbelts at the time of the crash.

Your partner quickly evaluates the ejected passenger. The patient, a 20-year-old male, hit a concrete retaining wall after being ejected. He sustained a catastrophic open head injury and is in cardio/respiratory arrest. Your partner notes brain matter and blood coming from the man's nose, mouth and ears, as well as a large defect in his skull, and quickly deems this a mortal injury. He decides not to attempt resuscitation.

Your patient, a 30-year-old male, complains of back and chest pain. He describes the back pain, located exactly between his shoulder blades, as worse than the chest pain. He also has slight shortness of breath, with bruising over his sternum and epigastric area, but none on his back.

While your partner obtains this patient's vital signs and places him on high-flow oxygen via non-rebreather mask, you obtain a complete history. *Vital signs:* pulse 110, blood pressure 178/100 and respiratory rate 30.

The patient claims he has no pertinent medical history and denies taking any medications. The police tell you the vehicle was traveling at about 55 mph when your patient lost control and skidded off the road, striking the pole. The steering column is bent. You find a pulse in both arms, but femoral pulses are diminished. His relatively high BP strikes you as odd for a trauma patient. You rapidly extricate him from the vehicle.

By this time, the BLS unit has arrived on scene and offers to take your patient to the hospital so you can go back in service. You decide to remain with the patient because of the associated fatality, mechanism of injury and his elevated BP. You start a large-bore IV of normal saline at a keep-vein-open rate while en route to the trauma center.

On your arrival at the ED, the trauma team begins assessing the patient and hears your presentation. The surgeon quickly examines him and requests an ultrasound of the chest. The results show an aortic rupture, so blood is ordered STAT, and he's whisked off to the bright lights and cold steel of the operating room—all within 15 minutes.

Discussion
Later, you learn your patient survived an injury that carries an 80–90% mortality rate in the first hour. The surgeon tells you that overhydration and further BP increases might have prompted complete rupture and lethal bleeding within the chest.

Traumatic aortic rupture usually results after falls from great heights and high-speed MVAs. These forces on the body's trunk cause the aorta to partially tear where it attaches to the chest wall. Sometimes (as with this patient), the outer layer of the artery remains intact, allowing for repair in the operating room. Other times, it's completely severed, and the patient dies quickly.

Chest and back pain prove the most common presentations. Patients often describe the back pain as worse. This patient's BP was so high because the injury basically shut off half the blood supply to the lower body. The bleeding within the vessel's lumen compresses the artery. This subsequently increases flow to the arms and upper body and reduces flow below the injury site—not an uncommon finding in aortic ruptures.

Conclusion

Patients often have such occult and perilous conditions that we may wish they had an early warning system flashing on their body to alert us to their problem. An early warning system does exist. It's called knowledge and clinical judgment. Listen to your inner voice, and let it guide your decisions.

3
CARDIAC EMERGENCIES

Rush to Judgment

"We judge ourselves by what we feel capable of doing;
others judge us by what we have done."
—Henry Wadsworth Longfellow

A colleague once told me emergency medicine is the art of making accurate decisions with incomplete information. The funny thing is, we occasionally set ourselves up for failure by believing information we suspect or know is false. Sometimes, we approach a patient with preconceived ideas, such as an emergency call at a nursing home. It's near the end of your shift, and you begin to think perhaps the assignment is not really an emergency at all. In cases like this, some of us—having made up our minds about the call and wanting our preconceived sentiments proved—may misinterpret straightforward patient presentations.

In busy services, this is especially apparent when dealing with cardiac arrest patients. As a rookie, I could not imagine a cardiac arrest could become routine with all the excitement, procedures, things to be done. But it happens. It may become routine, but as this case illustrates, we cannot allow ourselves to become complacent.

Scenario
One half-hour before shift change, your ALS ambulance is assigned to respond to a female in cardiac arrest. Immediately, your partner starts bitching about late assignments. The dispatcher tells you the patient's age is unknown. It takes about five minutes to arrive on scene. As you pull up, you notice the BLS vehicle turning the corner at the same time. From the fourth floor window, the police call down to you that the patient is a DOA. The system you practice in allows on-scene pronouncement and allows you to evaluate the patient and (should you determine that they do not require ALS) release the patient to the EMTs. Your partner informs the EMTs the pronouncement is theirs and places your vehicle back in service.

For obvious reasons, the EMTs are not the happiest folks in the world at this point. As you drive toward the garage and quitting time, the EMTs call for paramedics to respond to a cardiac arrest at the location you just left. Many things cross your mind. *Among the most notable:* embarrassment that this is something your partner and you will need to explain, anger that the BLS crew cannot get a simple DOA pronouncement right and a little optimism that this is a screw-up by the cops or EMTs. None of these proves to be the case.

On your return, you find the EMTs doing CPR on a 40-year-old woman they are moving to the ambulance. They tell you they defibrillated this lady with the AED twice; she regained a pulse for about a minute and then lost it. The AED did not indicate a shockable rhythm at that point, and the patient was moved to the vehicle. You and your partner suppress thoughts of damage control and your reputation as you try to get this lady breathing again. You work on her feverishly until you get to the hospital. Interestingly, the thought of getting home on time doesn't seem so important now. The patient arrives at the hospital pulseless and is pronounced dead shortly thereafter.

As you reflect on the patient and your actions, the cause of the cardiac arrest is inconsequential. You and your partner grapple with many questions as you discuss the case. Would this patient have survived with your ALS intervention from the beginning? What about her family? What about your job, your reputation?

Were there mistakes here? Sure! In your rush to end the tour, your partner told the BLS crew to handle the DOA pronouncement. Fine, if one or both of you had seen and pronounced the patient and then let the EMTs handle the paperwork. (Note this is the best situation in the world—where I come from, you pronounce *and* do the paperwork.) *The problem here:* Since you really didn't want to do the assignment, you took the police officer's word the patient was dead as a legitimate excuse to get back for the tour change.

Questions about the patient's possible outcome with earlier ALS intervention will remain open, because no one will ever know. Local procedures and supervisory personnel will resolve questions about your actions and possible consequences. Your professional reputation is something that, in a large part, your attitude will determine. We all make mistakes. The successful among us learn from them and avoid repeating them. The choice is yours.

More than Meets the Eye

"You can observe a lot by just watching."—*Yogi Berra*

EMS students often claim skills are the most enjoyable part of their classes. They take great pride in their prowess in applying backboards, getting the tube or dropping the line. But the truth is these psychomotor skills require very little brain power. They're like shaving. When was the last time you had to stop to read the directions on a can of shaving cream? It's a skill, and once you've done it enough, you barely need to think about it.

The real brain power of EMS work is in patient assessment. I would much rather hear a student say, "I nailed the assessment of that patient" than, "I got four tubes in the OR yesterday." Assessment is truly the art form of what we do, and without it we would be lost in trying to decide which protocols and procedures we should use. So why would students rather spend their time in skill practice than doing sample assessments?

Skill practice is easier and perhaps more straightforward than the thinking process needed for assessment. But you wouldn't be reading this if you were just looking for easy, so let's see what you think of this patient.

Scenario

The call is to the bedside of a hard-of-hearing, 75-year-old nursing home resident who is complaining of neck and upper abdominal pain. Communication is difficult. The man's hearing aid does not seem to work, and a lot of shouting in his ear is necessary to be heard. The man shouts back that he's been hurting for four to six hours. He denies any respiratory difficulty, is alert, and his skin is cool and dry. His vital signs are BP 98/60, pulse 60, and his respiratory rate is 20. Pupils are equal and reactive, conjunctiva are pale, lung sounds are clear, the belly is soft and nontender. The rest of the physical exam is unremarkable.

A tired-looking LPN tells you the man has been fairly healthy, although he does have a 15-year history of insulin-controlled diabetes, and he suffers from rheumatoid arthritis for which he takes Indocin 50 mg/day. He has no history of cardiac problems or hypertension, and he doesn't drink alcohol or smoke.

Nothing seems to have provoked the pain, and it remains constant. Nothing makes it better or worse (not even palpation). The patient characterizes the pain as "hurting like hell, in my stomach and neck." You ask him to characterize the pain on a severity scale of 1 to 10, but after shouting the question several times, you give up. From the grimace on his face and his grunts, you can tell he has significant pain.

During the exam, the man shouts that he is beginning to feel lightheaded and nauseated. His color remains good, but when vitals are repeated a slightly slower pulse and lower blood pressure is found (P 48, BP 80/60).

What are your impressions? First, are you jaded by the nursing home sick call and the difficulty in communicating with the man? My feeling is that most of us tend to have biases when it comes to emergency responses to these facilities. Is this bad? It is if it affects your assessment. It's tempting to take the vague symptoms of the elderly without much regard, especially if the attending staff is less than enthusiastic and communication with the patient is difficult. The idea here is to be aware that the bias may cloud our assessment.

Now, what is this patient's problem? Is this just a stiff neck and a belly ache? As Sigmund Freud once said, "Sometimes a cigar is just a cigar." Does the fact that the patient is elderly factor into your decisions here? What about the diabetic and arthritis history? Perhaps the abdominal pain is a reaction to the arthritis medications? Or is something more ominous going on here? At this point we can't be sure, so let's treat what we see and keep going.

As we observed, the patient is now lightheaded and nauseated, and having some changes in vital signs. So what are the correct BLS interventions? With the hypotension and the slow heart rate, we'll want to start some high-flow oxygen, help this gentleman to a comfortable position, keep an eye on his vitals and oops! here comes ALS.

What should ALS be doing? Besides listening to the excellent BLS assessment, we'll be hooking up the monitor and, oh my, look what we find (see ECG strip, next page). Clearly we have a third-degree heart block and as they say, it's show time. Now it's time to flex those skills. We need to start an IV, check vitals again, rev up the pacemaker and think about administering some atropine, all while we prepare to transport this gentleman to the ED.

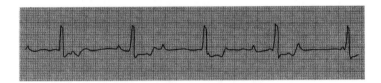

Case discussion
This patient's chief complaint was of neck and upper abdominal pain—not a typical presentation for someone having a heart attack. However, with a history of diabetes, all bets are off! Diabetics have been known to have MIs with little or no chest pain. But it's not just diabetics.

Recent data also indicates that women and elderly patients are also more likely to have atypical presentations. And then there's the age thing. Only 45% of patients over age 85 have chest pain as a complaint with myocardial infarction. These patients may or may not have shortness of breath or abdominal pain, or anxiety.

Remember CPR training when we taught the symptoms of a heart attack. What did we tell people to look out for? The distinct chest and/or neck, and/or jaw pain (perhaps a toothache), shortness of breath, sweating or nausea. We often taught these as a cluster but remember, the patient only needs one of these symptoms. Thus, you can see the importance of the patient interview and history. The initial vital signs seemed stable enough. However, during the interview, the patient began to get nauseated and syncopal, indicating poor perfusion, probably as a result of his bradycardia. Thus the patient's greatest need is for therapeutic interventions that will increase his heart rate.

These modalities are reflected in the ALS interventions. Pacing is the preferred method of increasing heart rate in this case. The use of analgesics/sedatives (morphine, diazepam) are recommended in alert patients because of the fact that transthoracic pacing is often uncomfortable. Atropine is a second-line agent in this case because of the fact that it cannot be depended upon to increase the heart rate in this rhythm (third-degree heart block).

The rest of the call proceeds without event. Upon arrival at the ED, your patient is evaluated and an ECG is done. The physician informs you that the cardiogram demonstrated an inferior wall myocardial infarction. She goes on to explain that such infarctions frequently present with abdominal pain, nausea, vomiting, bradycardias and hypotension. The patient's hospitalization is uneventful, and he is discharged 10 days later with a permanent pacemaker and a new battery in his hearing aid.

The bottom line here is recognizing that our patients are our clients. That's right, I said it! Clients. The sooner we realize this, the sooner we will catch up to other public service organizations, like the phone company, who used to refer to me as a "rate payer," and now calls me Mr. Werfel, valued customer. Our clients deserve our full attention and appropriate care and that is best expressed in performing a thoughtful, thorough and systematic assessment. Think about it.

Lulled by Machinery

"Technology: The knack of so arranging the world that we need not experience it."—Max Frisch

I have just finished reading one of those hefty EMS product catalogues. I was amazed at the hundreds of products now available for EMS providers—plastic backboards, gloves, stethoscopes, collars and piles of new computer-driven electronic devices. I counted no less than four different pulse oximeters and scores of high-tech diagnostic and treatment tools—all designed to improve patient care. Although I'm pleased the profession has progressed to the point where manufacturers now make clear efforts to cater to our perceived prehospital needs, I have rather mixed feelings about these gadgets. It now seems that the only real view we have of our patients is through the connection of some technological device (we obtain with a toll-free telephone number and a credit card). What happened to the old trusty methods of listening, touching and observing? It's telling that among all the items listed there were only three textbooks advertised. In my humble opinion, these devices have about as much to do with ensuring good patient care as one's choice of a pen or pencil does to ensure a best seller! How do I reach this shocking conclusion? Let's peruse the following interesting case.

Scenario

A BLS unit is called to a private doctor's office for a 50-year-old female with "difficulty breathing." When the EMT-Ds arrive on scene, they find a frightened frantic physician telling them, "I shocked her out of V-tach! You guys gotta get her to the hospital." The EMT-Ds call for a paramedic backup and continue into the office with their equipment. The woman, attached to a big old cardiac monitor/defibrillator, is alert and oriented, and as the EMT-Ds begin their assessment of the woman, the physician impatiently begins to shout the conflicting message that they need to get moving with the patient now, but that he "will not let the patient go anywhere without a damned cardiac monitor!"

You can imagine the pressure such a situation places on the providers. Both the physician and the patient are customers and both have valid needs. The providers want to do what's right. The crew chief remembers that the semi-automatic external defibrillator they were recently issued has, as one of its features, an LCD monitor screen built in. In an effort to expedite transport of the woman and calm the physician, the EMT-Ds put the defib pads on the patient and turn on the SAED. This initially calms the doctor, but as he examines the displayed ECG he starts shouting "she's back in V-tach!" But rather than cardiovert again, he orders the crew to get the patient to the nearest hospital.

The BLS crew packages the patient and begins the drive to the receiving hospital 10 minutes away. The crew member interviewing the patient finds an alert and lucid 50-year-old complaining of palpitations and nausea. The vital signs are: BP–100/70, pulse–120, RR–20. She has no medical history or medications. She claims that "it hurt like hell when the doc put those paddles on me."

Halfway to the hospital the EMTs are met by the responding medic fly car. The medic gets aboard the ambulance and looks at the ECG monitor on the SAED and exclaims "Oh my God, she's in V-tach!" and then he presses the "analyze" button. The software-driven voice advises the crew to stand back, that it is analyzing the rhythm. It then tells them that a shock is indicated and it begins charging. The increasing beeping of the charging capacitor reaches a crescendo and the electronic voice says "Shock patient" as the display indicates 200 joules. The paramedic then informs the patient that "she will feel a little shock."

By now you are shaking your head in disbelief. So was I as I later listened to the medic's voice on the cassette tape that was activated on the SAED at the beginning of the incident. The paramedic then proceeded to shock this poor lady no less than six times, after which the patient, having resisted all attempts to do her in, remained quite alert in her V-tach, and was transported to the hospital. Once in the ED, the woman was treated appropriately for her dysrrhythmia and made (thank God) an uneventful recovery.

What do you think about this case? Without a doubt, some of you are appalled that someone can really screw up this bad! You are probably wondering why we are talking about this case. Is it not just a simple case of negligence in which the BLS crew should be disciplined and the medic fired? Perhaps, but I'm not so sure we should dismiss this case so easily. Upon examination we will find that major errors of this type are actually made up of several smaller, more benign, errors. Of mistakes, Pearl S. Buck once said, "Every great mistake has a halfway moment, a split second when it can be recalled and perhaps remedied." Let's examine these errors in detail:

In my humble opinion, gentle reader, the SAED should never have been purchased (or for that matter made) with the monitor as an accessory. It would seem to me that if a device is going to be used only for resuscitation of pulseless/apneic folks, the monitor is, at best, something else to malfunction or, at worst, as we see, an invitation to near-disaster.

AEDs should only be placed on an apneic-pulseless patient ... period! Clearly the crew was led to do something that was contrary to their training by either an upset physician or (as I hope) their innate desire to help this patient. The BLS crew should have been much more assertive with the physician but as many of us know, one of the most difficult calls to manage can be the one in a medical clinic–especially when the patient is critical and the physician frightened.

Now we get to the actions of the paramedic. As I said, the medic was heard clearly on the tape telling the patient that she was going to feel the shock several times! Most of you will probably agree when I say that I have never had to tell a patient to prepare themselves for a defibrillation. By definition these patients are either in ventricular fibrillation or pulseless ventricular tachycardia. These rhythms are quite incompatible with life. Our instructors told us years ago that if the patient was talking to you while the monitor indicated an arrest rhythm, you had better evaluate them further. The paramedic made a huge mistake, but we can see this situation began honestly with the EMT-Ds wanting to help the patient in the doctor's office, but once they deviated from protocol by placing the AED on a patient with a pulse a chain reaction was put in place.

Why didn't the paramedic stop the incident? What was he thinking? He had the appropriate protocols for the treatment of this patient, and these protocols included the administration of medications and, if necessary, electrical cardioversion. Then why did this happen? A momentary lapse in which he confused the two distinct algorithms for V-tach and decided to act without attaching his monitor/defibrillator? I'm sure we'll never fully know, but there is a big lesson here. We need to be aware that technology will never replace a caring, vigilant human being overseeing patient care. The computerization of our profession is in its infancy, and it's important to realize that total reliance on a machine or device can lead us down a treacherous path. Medical devices are neither good nor bad and they help patient care but only when their use is overseen by thoughtful, seeing, touching and listening providers. We must guard against being lulled into thinking that our machines and electronics can exercise that exquisitely difficult-to-teach thing that we call clinical judgment.

Act Now

"To make no mistakes is not in the power of man, but from their errors and mistakes the wise and good learn wisdom for their future."—Plutarch

Is it possible to be so afraid of committing errors that we do nothing—the idea being that if we don't act, then we can't be accused of acting incorrectly?

Scenario

An EMT-D ambulance crew is dispatched to a grocery store to treat a male with chest pain. On arrival, the crew finds the store owner, a 48-year-old male, complaining of "squeezing" chest pain with shortness of breath. The patient tells Nancy, a crew member, that "it feels as though someone is squeezing my chest." The results of Nancy's primary survey: The patient is alert and talking, respirations are shallow at a rate of 24, radial and carotid pulses are palpable and rapid, and there are no obvious wounds or exsanguinating hemorrhage. His skin is cool and clammy. While Nancy documents the patient's history, her partner places him on high-flow oxygen and records the vital signs as pulse 120 and irregular, BP 110/60 and respirations 26. A head-to-toe survey reveals that the patient's pupils are equal and reactive to light; lung sounds are clear bilaterally; and there are no abnormalities found during examination of the abdomen, pelvis and back. The pulse oximeter indicates an O_2 saturation of 95% on room air.

The patient has a Novocain allergy. He isn't taking prescribed or over-the-counter medications and denies cardiac or other history. *His only hospitalization:* hernia surgery five years ago.

As mentioned in the chief complaint, the pain is of a "squeezing" quality and does not radiate or change with position or respiration. He tells Nancy that the chest pain and shortness of breath started approximately three hours earlier while he was doing inventory and that he has never had an episode of chest pain or difficulty breathing before. He says his pain rates a nine out of 10 in severity. Nothing makes the pain better or worse. The patient then tells Nancy that he is becoming nauseous and feels as though he is about to vomit.

At this point, Nancy's crew requests ALS assistance, but is informed that ALS is unavailable. So they place the patient in the ambulance and begin transport to the hospital. During transport the patient has a seizure, becomes cyanotic and pulseless. While starting CPR, the crew attempts to attach the semi-automatic defibrillator. After placing two well-adhering electrodes on the chest and pressing the "analyze" button, one of the crew realizes that the microcassette in the recording module is missing. While the crew chief decides what to do, the AED indicates a shockable rhythm. The crew chief elects not to shock the patient because of the absence of the microcassette. CPR is performed until arrival at the hospital (approximately eight to 10 minutes).

At the hospital, the patient's pulse and respiratory function are restored. He regains consciousness the next day, but has significant lapses of memory and violent outbursts during his hospitalization due to prolonged cardiac arrest. He is discharged several weeks later and placed on medication to minimize the outbursts.

Some may say that by knowingly using a machine that could not record the incident, Nancy and crew were exposing themselves to liability. If I were in that same situation, I would rather explain why I used the AED than why I decided against it.

What is the alternative? The only thing that works for a patient in ventricular fibrillation is the defibrillator. I've never seen a cardiac arrest victim regain pulse and consciousness by having an endotracheal tube placed or by having an IV line established.

There has been a protracted debate in some circles about defibrillators on aircraft. Some feel that having "only a stewardess" or other flight crew member using the defibrillator is inappropriate. (Some medics felt the same way when EMT defibrillation was proposed.) For me, the equation is simple: You are at 35,000 feet above the Atlantic and are in ventricular fibrillation—what is the alternative? What would you rather have in your bag of tricks? CPR until the plane lands (perhaps hours) or the defibrillator? Real tough choice. If it's me on that plane in V-fib, please have the flight attendant, pilot or person in the next seat use the defibrillator.

The unfortunate case of the 48-year-old grocer is no different. The net effect of 10 minutes of cardiac arrest on one's brain is the same, whether you're on a transatlantic flight that has no available defibrillator or in an ambulance where a decision is made not to use one. The choice is yours.

Appointment in Samarra

"Living is temporary; death is recorded in stone."
—*Anonymous*

One day a man who lived in Baghdad rushed to see the Grand Vizier. He wanted the Vizier's permission to go immediately to the town of Samarra. When the Vizier asked him why he was in such a rush, the man explained that he had seen the face of death in a dream. Death told him they would meet that night. "But," said the man, "if I ride swiftly, I will not be here tonight. I will be far away in Samarra." And so he fled.

That night the Grand Vizier dreamed and saw the face of death, and Death said to him, "Do not be afraid, for I am not concerned with you. Tonight, I have an appointment in Samarra."

This case helps us examine what transpired during one patient's appointment with old man death and his scythe.

Scenario

In the home stretch of your tour of duty, the dispatcher assigns your unit to a priority-one assignment: an "adult male, cardiac arrest, in front of Wayrich Industrial Sewage Systems, 144 First Ave. off Gregory Blvd. Time is now 1403."

En route, you tune your radio to the frequency of the police sector to which you are responding. On scene, the sector car confirms that CPR is in progress on a 55-year-old male. "Jeez," you think, "it has only been a month since we trained the cops in CPR and automated external defibrillation." Apparently, they're putting the equipment and training to good use.

The cops are performing rescuer CPR, and the AED is attached to the patient. But the officers tell you that the AED advised "no shock indicated." As you direct the cops to continue CPR, you perform an endotracheal intubation and your partner attaches the ECG and starts an IV. The patient appears to be in asystole—a rhythm you fondly refer to as "the ultimate bradycardia."

While an epinephrine bolus is administered, you quickly review the patient's physical presentation. His neck veins are flat, and you notice a telltale bulge under the patient's left clavicle. The patient has an implanted pacemaker. You've seen this before—pacemaker failure. "Outstanding," you think cynically. "Pacing is the best treatment available for a flat-line rhythm, and this guy's heart isn't responding to it."

Initially, your hunch is that this case will end up the same way as the other pacemaker failure cases you've treated; the patient will be pronounced dead. But then you remember something you read recently in a continuing education (CE) article and ask the crew to place the patient on his left side. They do so and suddenly you feel a pulse in the patient's carotid at a rate of 72. The patient begins to breathe on his own, and you see complexes on the ECG monitor. As you roll the patient onto his back, he again loses his pulse and becomes apneic. The grim reaper must be in a playful mood. Remembering an old football coach's rule that if a play works, run it again, you roll him on his side again. Once more, he regains his pulse and begins breathing on his own.

You maintain the patient in this position for the duration of the ride to the ED, realizing from the CE article that pacemaker wires sometimes detach from the patient's ventricle and can float down and reinsert themselves when a patient is placed on their left side. On arrival, the patient is still breathing, has a pulse and is slowly regaining consciousness. He is rapidly moved from the ED to the cardiac catheterization lab to fix the problem. Another life saved.

We all have our own appointments in Samarra. In fact, an EMS career places you face-to-face with death time and again. One of the purposes of our training is to forestall this event for as long as possible. Although we possess many high-tech weapons for use in this fight, sometimes just using our brains works better.

Although we can't always keep the grim reaper from reaching Samarra, we can hide his car keys and delay his arrival for a while. Learning from a CE article that dislodged pacemaker wires can sometimes be floated back into position is a valuable piece of knowledge. Applying it in the field to save a patient's life is priceless.

Avoid Assessment Traps

"Doctors can bury their mistakes, but architects can do little more than advise their clients to plant ivy."
—*Frank Lloyd Wright*

Students in EMS classes often complain about the written examinations. They commonly call the questions poorly written, vague or just plain confusing. The one question type universally condemned is a case presentation that progresses through several steps. It usually goes something like this:

Question 1: Your patient complains of X, Y and Z. What do you think is wrong with the patient?

Question 2: Based on your decision in question 1, what is the most appropriate intervention?

Question 3: Based on your decision in question 1 and your treatment in question 2, what should you do next for your patient?

You get the idea. The students complain that if they make an assessment error, all subsequent answers will be incorrect. It's unfair, they claim. Do their assertions hold water? Let's examine this case to find out.

Scenario

Today you're working with Roy Gilbert, someone you graduated from paramedic school with a couple of years ago. As you both reminisce about the class and where your various colleagues are, the dispatcher sends you to "a 60-year-old female asthmatic, 666 Jules Road. The corner of Donelan Blvd. Time out is 1005."

The dispatcher also sends a BLS unit to back you up. Outstanding, you think, because the BLS crews now carry albuterol and nebulizers for an asthma pilot program.

Your vehicle arrives on scene ahead of the EMTs. You find a 60-year-old female who is slightly lethargic and breathing rapidly. Her husband tells you she had some abdominal pain prior to complaining of shortness of breath. *The patient's vitals:* pulse 90, respirations 28, blood pressure 88/70. You hear wheezing when you listen to her lungs. Her skin is cool, clammy and ashen. She continues to complain of abdominal pain. In addition to her asthma history, she tells you she's a diet-controlled diabetic and had a heart attack seven years ago.

When you ask the husband for his wife's medications, he returns with the ubiquitous shoebox. The patient takes prescribed albuterol via nebulizer and completed two treatments prior to your arrival, without relief.

Roy places the patient on oxygen and prepares to give her a metaproterenol treatment because he feels it's clearly an asthma attack. He repeats the vital signs and obtains a 12-lead ECG. It demonstrates Q waves and S-T elevation in leads II, III and AVF. Acute inferior wall myocardial infarction (MI): The picture clicks for you—cardiogenic shock. You immediately discontinue the metaproterenol and request a dopamine drip. You transport the patient, and she's admitted to the coronary care unit.

Assessment clues
You ask the ED physician about the case. She reminds you that cardiogenic shock carries a mortality of 70–90%, even when the patient is hospitalized. It's caused by a decrease in the heart's pumping capacity. The most common cause of cardiogenic shock is MI, which results when dead heart muscle tends not to contract. She informs you that infarcts of the inferior wall of the left ventricle will more likely cause shock than other locations. When cardiogenic shock manifests, 40% of the heart is probably involved.

She goes on to say that physical exam of the cardiogenic shock patient will reveal a person in the midst of an MI with the usual symptoms, including chest pain, shortness of breath and signs of pulmonary edema and diaphoresis. In this case, the patient had abdominal pain. This may be due to the patient's history of diabetes (which changes the pattern and intensity of the pain) or the fact that women often have atypical MI presentation.

The complaint that led you furthest astray was the wheezing. If she had crackles, you insist, the two of you would have zeroed in on the problem faster. The doctor tells you to remember that in the early stages of pulmonary edema, patients often present with the wheezes of cardiac asthma. You both mentally file the lesson for future reference.

Lessons learned
Obtain and process as much information as possible and make informed decisions within the purview of your protocols and scope of practice, avoiding the myopia

that accompanies those driven by protocol alone. On the written exam questions referenced earlier, once you decide on a problem and a route of treatment, you change your approach at your own peril. In practice, not changing treatment when other facts and information become available may imperil your patient. It's a sobering thought and an important point to remember.

Fatally Forgotten

*"Not the power to remember, but its very opposite,
the power to forget, is a necessary condition
for our existence."* —*Sholem Asche,* The Nazarene

Have you ever forgotten something? Your anniversary?
Valentine's Day? Forgot to pick your kids up from
school? I'm sorry to say I forget where I parked my car
at work more often than I care to report. It's actually
amazing that I can retain so much arcane EMS information and still forget a mundane item like where I parked
my car. I guess we've all forgotten things.

But what about forgetting something of importance
to a patient? Can it happen? Sure. Does it have to be a
big thing to have a catastrophic result? Let's examine this
case to find out.

Scenario

You're working a day shift with your regular partner,
Gerard. As you drink a cappuccino and work on the

Sunday *New York Times* crossword, the dispatcher's tones shake you out of your daydream. "A 40-year-old male complaining of chest pains. *Location:* Scott residence, 505 Marilyn St., corner of Bourne Ave. Time out is 1422."

As you push the "en route" button on the data terminal, you go through a mental checklist of problems this guy might have. What equipment will you bring in? What kind of access to the patient will you have? How many flights of stairs will you have to climb to reach the patient?

On arrival, you see a woman running out of her home. She screams that her husband, unconscious and not breathing, was awake and alert just a minute ago and then passed out and stopped breathing.

You and your partner quickly go into the house and to the patient's side. His color is still good. You tell your partner it looks like this guy just went down. You both know you have the best results resuscitating witnessed or quickly discovered arrests.

You get the defibrillator paddles and move the "lead" switch to "paddles." As you place the paddles on the victim's chest, your partner says the man has no pulse. You look at the ECG screen and see ventricular tachycardia. This now becomes a protocol-driven event.

You place the conductive pads on the victim's chest and charge the defibrillator to 200 joules. You deliver the shock and have your partner repeat a pulse check. No pulse. You shock the victim at 300 joules with no results and then again at 360 joules. Your partner successfully intubates the patient while you put the ECG electrodes on the chest and look at the monitor. You see a flat line. You've now shocked the victim into asystole.

The BLS crew who arrived to back you up starts

CPR. You establish an IV and administer epinephrine. However, there's no change in the patient's condition or ECG rhythm. You feel uncomfortable. Something in your mind tells you this guy should have a better rhythm. His color is pink, and he's being well-ventilated with 100% oxygen. There's still no pulse, and the patient's ECG still shows flat line—what your instructor called "the ultimate bradycardia."

You administer atropine and repeat the epinephrine, as you have every five minutes since the initial dose. You wish the patient were at least in fibrillation because you'd have some form of rhythm to work with. This patient has nothing going for him when you call medical control. The doctor orders more epinephrine and pacing. Neither changes his condition.

The physician orders dextrose and Narcan, but these drugs also prove ineffectual. You tell the doctor you've been on scene with this patient for 25 minutes, and he has not responded. She tells you to end your efforts and gives you a time of pronouncement.

The BLS crew stops CPR, and you have the difficult task of telling the woman that her husband did not survive. Her wails of grief pierce your ears as you go back into the room to clean up your equipment.

You remove the ET tube from the patient's trachea and pull the IV. Your partner takes the ECG electrodes off the man's chest and places the wires in the pouch attached to the machine. His face turns pale as he points to the defibrillator. Your eyes follow his finger to the lead switch. You feel a paroxysm of nausea. It's in the "paddles" mode.

The patient's real ECG never appeared on the monitor. Because the paddles only show the rhythm when they're on the chest, a flat line showed when you switched to the electrodes. This patient could have had a shockable rhythm throughout the event, and you never would have known it. As you try to take this all in, the crying gets louder.

Discussion
This is a terrible story to be sure, but the more chilling reality is that it could happen to any of us. In this case, the provider has a small memory lapse with catastrophic results. *The true challenge of EMS:* Trying to remember a multitude of facts and treatment modalities and do so without forgetting anything—big or small. In EMS, it's truly better to remember correct actions than spend a significant part of your life trying to forget the consequences of your errors.

Patient's Perspective

"A human being an ingenious assembly of portable plumbing." —*Christopher Morley,* Human Being

I bet if I polled EMS practitioners about their greatest fears, being a patient would show up consistently among the top answers. As EMS providers, we have a helper mentality. We come to the aid of the sick and injured. All our training is vectored toward this end. We find it truly unsettling to receive the care instead of providing it.

We sometimes deliver the most questionable care to our own colleagues. This is partly our fault—much of it is theirs. *Example:* Many years ago, the center fielder on my EMS agency's softball team fell hard during a game. Even though they heard him scream in pain and saw his obvious discomfort, other EMTs and paramedics urged him to walk off what turned out to be an ankle fracture. For a civilian with a similar injury, those providers would have immobilized the victim's entire leg. They wouldn't have taken any chances.

How do we react when we're the patients? Will everything be OK when we're the ones on the stretchers? Let's examine this case to find out.

Scenario

You're working a 3 p.m.–11 p.m. shift. The dispatcher assigns you to assist a "48-year-old male, sick; 334 Romano Blvd. between Arthur Ave. and Christian Lane. Time out is 1609."

As you proceed to the scene you remember the ubiquitous sick call can run the gamut of a headache to a cardiac arrest. You pull up, walk to the front door and find a patient with a familiar face. Mitch, a long-time paramedic, helped pique your interest in paramedicine. He's been a county police officer for more than 12 years and is now responsible for providing EMT and AED training to each class of police recruits.

He tells you that for the past six hours he's had left-side abdominal and rib pain. He says he believes that if he could belch, he would feel better. He denies any shortness of breath or diaphoresis.

Mitch is in great shape and ran three miles with the recruits two days ago. He says his cholesterol is below 200, and he doesn't smoke. He takes no medications and reports that heart trouble does not run in his family. In fact, his 82-year-old father remains in good health. He also says he's sure this incident isn't heart-related. He laughs and tells you he performed his own version of a stress test before he called EMS: He ran up and down the stairs several times, and the pain remained the same. If it were heart pain, he insists, it would have gotten worse. Right? (How many of you have pulled the same stunt?)

As you obtain a detailed history and complete your assessment, it becomes apparent the patient is trying to put the best light on his symptoms. When you ask about the duration of his chest pain, he corrects you and says it's abdominal pain—not chest pain. When you note that he is diaphoretic, he says it's because he ran up the stairs in a warm house, not because of his discomfort. You conclude that with the subtle distinctions between word meanings and his corrections, this incident has more similarities to the deposition of a former president than to a patient assessment.

You and your partner believe Mitch is experiencing GI-related pain. However, as precautionary measures, you administer oxygen, establish an IV and obtain a 12-lead ECG. The ECG shows a normal sinus rhythm at a rate of 100 with no changes. You transport the patient uneventfully to the University Medical Center.

When you check in on Mitch later in the shift, his ECG remains normal, and the ED physician says he believes the pain is GI-related. You go home secure in the fact that your mentor is in good hands and will probably be home sleeping before you are.

You return to work two days later and learn Mitch's cardiac enzymes came back high. An emergent cardiac cath showed narrowing in four coronary arteries. He had bypass surgery the next morning, which required 34 inches of his saphenous vein (a leg vein) to construct six bypass grafts.

Your entire crew, frightened out of the "It can't happen to me" mindset, seriously entertains the possibility of getting cardiac work-ups.

Discussion

What's the first thing heart attack patients experience? Denial. It's probably worse when an EMS provider is the patient. Although this case has a happy ending, it's easy to see how the ending might have been different. What if Mitch had continued to perform his home-brewed stress test?

We can't answer this question, but our experience lets us predict the outcome. Once again, vigilance and suspicion remain your best allies in all situations. Don't let a patient (or coworker) rationalize away good care. Conduct a complete assessment, and treat the symptoms as they present.

Myocardial Dilemma

"Elementary, My Dear Watson."
—*Sir Arthur Conan Doyle*, Adventures of Sherlock Holmes

Scenario

Dispatch sends your unit to a nursing home for a male with chest pain. On arrival, you're directed to the patient's bedside. Mr. Jackson, a gentleman of 80, complains of chest pain. He says the pain began about two hours ago and hasn't changed with position or breathing (chest movement). He describes it as a squeezing pain in the middle of his chest, radiating to his arm and jaw. He denies any shortness of breath or nausea. The patient also denies a heart history (which the staff corroborates) or any recent trauma that could have triggered the pain.

He admits to an ulcer history; he was hospitalized several years ago for a bleeding, perforated ulcer. The staff tells you he takes only Pepcid and has no known allergies. His skin is warm and dry, and he's alert and oriented x 3. You initially think the case may be a rule out

(R/O) myocardial infarction (MI). *Vital signs:* BP 98/72, pulse 54, regular ventilations at 20 and clear lung sounds.

Your partner runs a 12-lead ECG on the patient. It exhibits a sinus rhythm at 54, with deep Q waves and ST segment elevation evident in leads II, III and AVF. You administer high-flow oxygen via non-rebreather mask and start an IV. You and your partner now must decide on the therapy indicated for this patient. Why do you think it's a R/O MI? What's the significance of the ECG changes?

Although not everyone who complains of chest discomfort is aggressively treated as an MI, some clear cases sing out for prehospital intervention. This is one of those cases.

Why does this patient's complaint worry us? Because he's complaining of chest heaviness that doesn't change with movement or positioning. In fact, the pain radiates to his arm and jaw—a presentation highly suggestive of MI. However, other culprits could include pulmonary embolism (PE), thoracic aneurysm or ulcer pain.

You should always consider PE when a patient suffers chest discomfort. Chest pain that's pleuritic in nature strongly suggests PE. Additionally, you'd probably expect to see tachypnea, tachycardia and possibly hypotension and cyanosis in the PE patient. These symptoms weren't present here.

Could this be a thoracic or abdominal aneurysm? Probably not. Usually an aneurysm involves a male in their 50s or 60s. Although older folks do sometimes suffer aneurysms, the patient usually complains of a "ripping, tearing or boring" pain in the back. In addition, the vast majority of patients with aneurysms have long-standing hypertensive histories. Neither was present.

Could this be an ulcer? Again, probably not. Ulcer pain is usually of a gnawing nature and tends to change with position and meals. Although many other causes of chest discomfort exist, you should always consider the most likely cause and think of horses, not zebras, when you hear hoofbeats.

Deep Q waves and ST segment elevation in leads II, III and AVF are consistent with an inferior wall infarction. The posterior left coronary artery is most often involved, but the left circumflex or left coronary artery can sometimes be the culprit. Patients with this particular event are highly susceptible to heart blocks, bradycardia, hypotension and cardiogenic shock. Knowing this may help you maintain your vigilance of the patients' vital signs during treatment and transport.

Treatment options
Because patient apprehension and fear drive the myocardial oxygen demand upward and can actually increase an infarct's size, pain relief is vital for MI patients. Remember the ACLS bromide that "MONA (morphine, oxygen, nitroglycerin and aspirin) greets all patients"? The new ACLS guidelines recommend MONA for all patients with ischemic chest pain. Let's examine each aspect of MONA.

Morphine has about as many dosage recommendations as there are EMS practitioners. Most recommendations start with an initial dose in the range of 2–10 mg and repeat small doses of 2 mg every few minutes until the pain is relieved or side effects occur—namely respiratory depression and/or hypotension.

Although we know its analgesic and sedative effects, morphine also has beneficial hemodynamic properties. Morphine reduces the fluid load on the heart by acting as a vasodilator. This increased venous capacity decreases venous return and lowers blood pressure. *The upside:* The patient's myocardium has less work to do and, therefore, needs less oxygen.

Oxygen administration is indicated in all situations in which you might encounter hypoxemia. In giving patients oxygen, we increase alveolar oxygenation, resulting in increased hemoglobin saturation. This makes more oxygen available for the tissues. In these cases, give oxygen at high-flow rates. Monitor patients for improvement, as well as the respiratory depression that occasionally occurs in chronic obstructive pulmonary disease patients.

Nitroglycerin's potent vasodilatory effects reduce blood pressure and myocardial workload. In addition, this vasodilation affects (to a lesser degree) the coronary arteries, resulting in improved myocardial blood flow. The main concern with this drug is that many patients develop a tolerance to it. Obviously, don't give it to patients who have hypotension or elevated intracranial pressure.

Side effects include hypotension, tachycardia, dizziness and headache. Once exposed to air, nitroglycerin has a short shelf-life. It's light-sensitive, so store it in a dark place. Dosing is one 0.4 mg sublingual (SL) tablet or spray. You can repeat the dose every three to five minutes as required and as long as the patient maintains stable vital signs. The dose of nitroglycerin paste is usually one-half to one inch of ointment.

Aspirin blocks platelet aggregation and localized vasoconstriction by blocking a substance that causes the platelets to congregate (thromboxane A2). It has been demonstrated that administering aspirin early significantly reduces mortality in MI patients. Its only contraindication is known hypersensitivity. It can be used even if the patient has ulcer disease—if you decide the benefits outweigh the risks. The recommended dosage of aspirin is 160–325 mg. Patients need to chew the tablet for maximal beneficial effect, so use baby aspirin.

Finally, consider using a 12-lead ECG. Studies indicate that prehospital 12-leads may significantly reduce time to thrombolytic therapy and limit or reverse ischemic damage.

Case outcome
Under standing orders, you administer 0.4 mg SL nitroglycerin to the patient. He tells you that he's getting a burning sensation under his tongue. (This assures you of the drug's potency). In addition, as your partner retakes vitals, Mr. Jackson tells you that he's getting a headache. The patient's heart rate increases to 78. Both can be expected with nitroglycerin administration. The patient's blood pressure remains unchanged.

After confirming the patient is not allergic to aspirin (and taking the patient's ulcer into consideration), you administer 160 mg baby aspirin, also under standing orders.

You obtain another set of vitals. He demonstrates no change. You contact medical control and request a repeat of the SL nitroglycerin, a half inch of nitropaste and 2 mg morphine sulfate with repeat doses every five minutes until the chest pain is relieved or as long as the vital signs remain stable. The physician agrees.

The patient's vital signs remain stable as you begin transport. En route, Mr. Jackson tells you his pain has diminished substantially, so you discontinue medication.

On arrival at the hospital, the history, physical and ECG indicate an inferior wall infarct. The ED staff hustles the patient to the interventional cardiology lab to perform a cardiac bypass surgery. The patient has an uneventful recovery and is discharged several days later.

This case is a prime example of how a crew used their knowledge and experience to zero in on and treat a patient's problem. Use every case as a learning experience and don't forget to pass along those experiences to others. A member of your family might be the next chest pain patient they encounter.

Eternal EMS Vigilance

"Experience teaches slowly, at the cost of mistakes."

—James Frode

Have you ever made an error while working on a patient? Most (or all) of us have—your humble narrator included. A majority of those errors were probably minor: perhaps forgetting to document a finding or not following specific equipment-use directives. Although such errors don't happen regularly, many EMS providers have come to accept them as normal. I fervently disagree with accepting mistakes as the cost of doing business, but you can read this case and form your own opinion.

Scenario
It's finally fall. Summer's heat and humidity have abated, and all seems well with the world—then dispatch interrupts your calm. "Unit 13, respond for an adult male, sick at Jay Gardens Psychiatric Hospital, Arline Road and Stern Street. Time out is 1203." The in-vehicle com-

puter indicates your patient is a 50-year-old male employee complaining of abdominal pain.

On arrival, your partner takes vitals while you size up the patient. He says he's had abdominal pain for the past day or so and identifies the lower left abdomen as the location of his most severe pains. He tells you he vomited for the first time about an hour ago, but appears well nourished. He's alert and oriented x 3, and seems to be in no immediate distress. He denies experiencing any chest pain or shortness of breath. He takes no medications, doesn't smoke and reports no significant medical history.

His vitals: pulse 90, respirations 12 and BP 140/84. He has equal, reactive pupils and doesn't have pale conjunctivas. He has no jugular vein distention. His 12-lead ECG shows sinus rhythm at 90, with no ectopy or ischemic changes. Capillary refill takes one second, and the patient doesn't have orthostatic (positional) changes when you sit him up. The abdomen is soft and minimally tender in the left lower quadrant with no rebound tenderness.

In keeping with good medical practice, you administer high-flow oxygen via non-rebreather mask. Your protocols allow you to place an IV or heparin lock in the patient. You elect to go with the heparin lock.

You insert it and inject 2 mL of saline drawn from an ampule in the drug kit. (The heparin lock model you use requires you to inject 2 mL of normal saline into the device after placement.)

As you tape down the device and prepare the patient for transport, he suddenly complains of chest pain and shortness of breath. His pulse is now 200, and he's cyanotic.

Suddenly, the patient seizes and becomes pulseless and apneic. You start CPR, intubate the patient and begin rapid transport. Your efforts prove unsuccessful.

At the hospital, the ED physician says, "Sometimes this happens. Folks die, and we just happen to be witnesses."

You go back to your vehicle to straighten things up. You place a new heparin lock in the drug case and look for the open sterile saline ampule so you can replace it. You pick up the open ampule and read the label. Suddenly, your stomach churns, and you feel faint. The label doesn't say "Sterile Saline for Injection—5 mL." It says "Dopamine 800 mg/5 mL."

You quickly do the math—a maximum therapeutic dose of dopamine is 20 mcg/kg/minute. Assuming a large man, a maximum therapeutic dose for him might be 2,000 mcg per minute (20 mcg x 100 kg). You administered 320,000 mcg—160 times the therapeutic amount—in the second it took to inject it, your patient died from a catastrophic medication error. This story doesn't have a happy ending for anyone.

Discussion

We're all familiar with the small errors we learn from and get past. But we're also familiar with the big mistakes that make us shudder. That's exactly what I did today when I heard about a child who was accidentally killed during an MRI.

As you know, an MRI uses a powerful magnet to obtain high-resolution images of internal structures. Patients and workers alike are instructed to leave all metal objects at the door. In this case, an oxygen tank was left in the room and became a projectile when the magnet was powered up. The tank flew to the center of the MRI unit, striking a fatal blow to the child's head.

These stories exemplify how a small error can lead to a catastrophe if ignored or missed. Someone once said the price of freedom is eternal vigilance. It's also the price of high-quality patient care.

4
RESPIRATORY EMERGENCIES

Haunting Words

"Adversity is a hard school, but its alumni are apt to shine."—Anonymous

In early January, I heard a news report about a woman and her daughter who are suing a national theme park. They claimed the haunted mansion was too frightening, with horribly disfigured and bloody people pursuing the guests while holding the requisite chain saws, clubs and such.

Most patrons attend these haunted attractions expecting the unexpected, just as those of us in EMS should expect a certain level of uncertainty. Each day brings with it the anticipation of the unpredictable, the hot assignment and the unknown. Every patient represents a challenge for us to conquer. Does this unpredictability have a down side? Let's check out this case and find out.

Scenario

You're working a 24-hour shift with Mary Jo, the best partner you've worked with. On this day, however, Mary

Jo is angry about her previous day's losses at a nearby casino.

The two of you talk about her losses during a lull between calls when the dispatcher summons: "Medic 111 respond to an elderly male having difficulty breathing. Old No. 7 Road, the Daniels' Farm. Time out 0301."

As you drive along the dark, empty country roads, you review what could be wrong with the patient and the roles you'll each take on arrival. Mary Jo reminds you that your previous five patients all had the flu. It seems as though everyone is sick these days.

On scene, you find your 76-year-old patient sitting on the edge of the bed complaining he can't catch his breath. His symptoms began when he went to the bathroom 25 minutes earlier. Although he appears in distress, the patient actively tells his spouse what clothes to bring to the hospital. He has some visible accessory muscle use, and rales and rhoncii are audible without the use of a stethoscope. His respiratory rate is 30; his heart rate is a weak radial at 110. The BP is 108/70. He has a history of diabetes, hypertension and three previous myocardial infarctions, but does not complain of chest pain. He had gone to the doctor earlier that day because he felt ill and was diagnosed with the flu and given a prescription for an antibiotic.

You place the patient on high-flow oxygen and a cardiac monitor, which shows sinus tachycardia at 110. Seeing the cardiac monitor in use, the patient's wife becomes concerned and asks you if her husband will be OK. You ease her fears by explaining you think her husband has the flu—just like the doctor said—and that he'll be fine. Meanwhile, Mary Jo prepares a 5.0 mg Ventolin nebulizer that she administers under standing orders.

You begin transport. As you drive toward the hospital, Mary Jo starts a second Ventolin treatment. With your partner's encouragement, the patient begins to control his respiratory rate, and he no longer sounds quite so congested.

When you reach the hospital, you ask the patient's wife a few more questions for your report and assure her that her husband will be fine. You send her to the waiting room and look for the nurse to sign your patient care report.

You walk into the treatment room to find the doctor struggling to intubate the patient. The tube goes in; the patient arrests. You assist the ED staff with the code, but the patient remains unresponsive and 20 minutes later is pronounced dead.

As the distraught wife comes to the bedside, you cannot bring yourself to look at her. She sobs, "But you told me it was the flu, and he'd be all right." Those words haunt you for the rest of your shift. You find out later that the patient had respiratory failure due to pneumonia that led to the cardiac arrest. The elderly can crash quickly, the doctor tells you, especially with the history of diabetes, heart trouble and hypertension this old guy had.

Despite our best efforts ...
Patients sometimes die in spite of our best efforts. When we see a patient with mortal injuries, we can prepare ourselves and help the patient's relatives prepare themselves. We do this with carefully chosen words: "We're hoping that he'll start breathing on his own again, but you must prepare yourself that it may not happen."

However, when we think a patient will do OK, and they unexpectedly die, we feel guilty about misleading the family. Did I leave my guard down? Did I miss something?

Subconsciously I always expect patients who are

awake and talking when they reach the ED to survive. It invariably rattles me if I learn they didn't make it. Expect it to rattle you, too.

When we're confronted with a sick patient who has a history of prior MIs, diabetes and hypertension and whose age works against them, don't make promises you can't keep. Your EMS training teaches you that elderly patients with multiple conditions are an EMS time bomb waiting for just the right condition to trigger it. Remain alert for these patients, and render good EMS care. Leave the speeches and promises to the politicians.

Variety—The Spice of Life?

"It does not take much strength to do things, but it requires great strength to decide on what to do."
—Elbert Hubbard

While waiting to board a flight recently, I was struck by the decision-making process now involved in buying a cup of coffee. You can order house blend, decaf, café mocha, espresso, decaf espresso, café latte or decaf café latte, among others. You can also order espresso with a shot of various liqueurs or flavors. All these selections come in a multitude of sizes with steamed whole, 1% or 2% milk. Regardless of the number of appealing options I had that day, it helped to recall that my basic decision was about coffee.

Similarly, remembering the basics of patient care can help you wade through the myriad of possibilities surrounding a complex medical incident.

Despite the complex equipment and technology we possess, we must remember that they have not altered the way our patients present. This paraphernalia should not distract us from the importance of basic patient care. Skillful assessment still requires us to address each individual. The same disease can present in different people with a multitude of varying symptoms.

Example: A patient's chest pain can result from many things, including a pulled muscle caused by coughing or a myocardial infarction (MI). This case is a good example of the importance of basic patient care.

Scenario

You and your partner, Ray, are dispatched to a "35-year-old female with chest pain, 101-02 Princi Street, corner of Rudolph Ave." During the response, the two of you think out loud. Ray bets on angina or MI, but insists that the age is wrong. You say, based on age, you believe the patient could have pleurisy or a simple musculoskeletal chest wall problem.

You arrive on scene to find a 35-year-old, well-nourished female who has complained of chest pain and shortness of breath for the past 20 minutes. Her pulse is 150, respiration 22 and BP 110/70. Her only history is that of a heart valve replacement four months previously.

As Ray places the oxygen and ECG electrodes on the patient, she suddenly becomes pale, unresponsive and pulseless. ECG shows pulseless electrical activity (PEA) at 90. You start CPR, move the patient to the ambulance and begin transport. En route, you place an IV of saline and administer resuscitation drugs. You notify the hospital to expect a patient in arrest. The patient arrives and ED staff begin aggressive resuscitation, with no positive result.

This case unnerves you and your partner. You both attend the morbidity/mortality conference, where you learn your patient died from a large pulmonary embolus

(PE). The ED director tells you the patient's artificial heart valve is probably to blame because the turbulent blood flow around the valve lends itself to clot formation.

Common causes of PE include long-bone fractures, pregnancy, trauma, oral contraceptives, lupus and anything else that causes blood to pool (e.g., prolonged bed rest or extended air travel).

Massive PE is a common cause of unexpected death, ranking second only to MI. Although there are at least 650,000 cases annually, most clinicians (physicians included) do not properly appreciate the extent of the problem because it remains unsuspected until autopsy in 80% of cases.

Good luck on finding a "classic" case. Although the classic presentation is shortness of breath (SOB), chest pain and coughing up blood, signs and symptoms vary and may also include abdominal or shoulder pain, wheezing, diaphoresis, syncope, fever, distended neck veins or cough.

The ED physician points out that of those who die from massive PE, about 60% have SOB, 17% have chest pain and 3% cough up blood. The upside for both of you is that you did everything you could for your patient. The doc reminds you that appropriate prehospital treatment consists of oxygen, ECG monitor, rapid transport and an IV of saline or Ringer's solution. You feel better, but aren't anxious to deal with another PE for a while.

Conclusions

They say that variety is the spice of life. The same variety that makes EMS such an attractive field can create difficult assessment problems. Does a magic PE protocol exist that would have saved this crew's patient? No. Remember that protocols, although comprehensive in many venues, remain outnumbered by illnesses and symptoms. And although our new equipment can and does save lives, we can't let it distract us.

Sometimes the best decisions we make are the fundamental ones—oxygen, monitor and transport. Don't ever forget the basics of patient care. They'll help you address the needs of your patients 90% of the time.

You Haven't Seen Them All!

"Habit will reconcile us to everything except change."
−*Charles Caleb Colton*

Remember when there were good and bad habits? Good habits were working hard, eating right and getting up early. Bad habits were smoking, drinking or taking drugs. Lately, it seems like the word habit is only used in reference to something bad. Perhaps this is because bad habits take less effort to maintain than the good ones. This is demonstrated in the prehospital venue by the obviously bad habit of neglecting to check out the ambulance at the start of a shift and the less-obvious habits that have a profound influence on patient care. Consider this case.

Scenario
Imagine you are one of the medics responding to this actual call for a "difficulty breathing." In a housing project, you find an obese 19-year-old woman breathing rap-

idly. She says her chest is "killing" her and she can't breathe. Between grunts and gasps, she says she has had right-sided chest pain for the past 30 minutes. The room is dim, but you think you notice some circumoral cyanosis.

The patient's boyfriend is hovering over her while smoking. After you convince him to put out his cigarette, he explains that he and the patient had a major dispute three hours ago about his purchase of a new motorcycle. Meanwhile, the patient gasps and screams that the pain feels "like a knife" and worsens every time she takes a breath. She has no pertinent medical history and has never had an episode like this before. Her heart rate is 136, BP is 100/70, and the respiratory rate is 30. Her only medications are birth control pills and a one-pack-a-day smoking habit.

As you begin to place the patient on oxygen, your partner, a senior medic with 12 years experience, pulls you aside and tells you, "There's no way we are going to give oxygen to this nonsense!" She says the patient is obviously a hyperventilating head case and needs to breathe into a paper bag or a nonrebreather mask without the oxygen attached. Being a new, relatively inexperienced medic, you acquiesce to the will of your partner, even though your instructors warned you not to withhold oxygen from anyone. Your partner puts a nonrebreather on the patient without oxygen in hopes that she will slow her breathing. But after 10 minutes, the pain persists, and the decision is made to transport her to the hospital.

As you load the patient, you notice her neck veins are bulging, she is coughing and is progressively becoming more cyanotic. You mention this to your partner, but she waves it off. Somewhere in your gut is a nagging doubt that you are really doing the right thing for this patient. As if to confirm your suspicion, the patient suddenly has a hypoxic seizure and becomes unresponsive. A moment later, she is pulseless and apneic. How could you have been so wrong? You go for the quick-look paddles, your partner goes for the tube, and together you begin a valiant attempt at resuscitation, but nothing works.

On arrival, the hospital continues the effort but finally a young ED physician calls it and suggests that the woman probably had a pulmonary embolus (PE). This is confirmed on autopsy. Pulmonary emboli affect more than 600,000 Americans per year and kill about 38% of them. The causes are: venostasis (prolonged bed rest or sitting), pregnancy, trauma, increases in blood coagulabilty (oral contraceptives), injury to the veins from fractures or surgery, and other diseases (heart failure, MI, atrial fibrillation, infections, COPD and diabetes). Symptoms include shortness of breath, pleuritic chest pain, tachycardia, hypotension, anxiety, cyanosis, distended neck veins, crackles, wheezes, cough and hemoptysis. Because these broad symptoms may fit into several diseases, it is important to suspect PE whenever there are risk factors or vague and otherwise unexplained respiratory or cardiac findings.

Now let me ask, is experience always a good thing to have? Certainly not in this case! The more experienced partner has probably seen dozens of these "hysterical female" cases and remembers a day when EMS practitioners were taught to have patients breathe into paper bags to help them. Experience often gives rise to habit; some good, some bad.

When folks apply to paramedic programs, they worry about not having enough experience. Well, from where I'm sitting, this is not such a bad situation. In fact, not having a pile of old habits is an enviable position. But what if you've been around for a while? How do we combat bad habits? A good start is to realize EMS is the wrong field to apply the old maxim, "you seen one, you seen 'em all."

Removing the Box from Assessment

"Beware that you do not lose the substance by grasping at the shadow."— *Aesop,* Fables

Have you noticed how many EMS educators teach their material in nice tidy little modules? There are lessons on environmental emergencies, lessons on cardiac emergencies, lessons on trauma—all in handy separate teaching blocks. These nice compartments are even broken down further into sections on adult problems, geriatric problems and pediatric problems. It all makes for easy organized teaching and learning, but if the teacher is not careful, the students leave with the impression that everything they see in the field will fit into some neat little compartment.

Unfortunately, working in a dynamic environment like EMS does not match this sort of training that places signs, symptoms and causes into rigid pigeonholes. People are not pigeons, and they no more fit our artificial categories than they would fit into a bird's nest. It's the exception rather than the rule to see a "textbook" case, and yet we often exert great energy trying to push the grid of what we've learned onto reality.

Medicine has long been considered both an art and a science, and I see no reason to define EMS any differently. The science of what we do is the application of research-proven treatment modalities, and these fit nicely into training modules. The art of what we do is the assessment of the patient's problem. And here is where we need to suspend our need to compartmentalize because real field problems will cross all compartments and categories as the following case demonstrates.

Scenario
Your ambulance is sent on a call for an "adult male with difficulty breathing." En route, you are thinking the problem will probably be heart- or COPD-related. Upon arrival, you find an alert, muscular 24-year-old man sitting on the edge of his bed complaining of feeling sick and having a difficult time breathing. His color is good, and with a brassy voice he tells you in complete sentences that he has been sick for a couple of days with a cough and stuffy nose. Tonight, however, his throat is "killing him," and he feels like he can't get a good breath.

While listening to him, you realize his voice is somewhat muffled, and he keeps wiping drool from his mouth and chin. He has no medical history, takes no medications and has not seen a doctor recently. You place him on high-flow oxygen and proceed with your head-to-toe exam.

His skin is hot and dry. His pupils are equal and reactive to light, and the conjunctiva are pink. His neck is unremarkable. Lung sounds are clear, and nothing abnormal is assessed in the chest, abdomen or pelvis. During the exam, you notice that the man continues to sit forward and occasionally seems to be struggling for breath. He seems truly frightened and irritated.

Well, what do you think is wrong with this young gentleman? One of the medics suspects the man might have epiglottitis, but his partner rolls her eyes and disagrees. "We all know epiglottitis is a childhood illness," she states authoritatively. And how does she know that? Because in her original training class and in all the refreshers since, the only mention of epiglottitis was in the pediatric section. What does such training translate to in the day-to-day practice of prehospital medicine? It proclaims loudly that adults do not get epiglottitis. But this is totally false, oh gentle reader. Adults do get epiglottitis, and in fact, adult presentation of epiglottitis may be on the rise. Furthermore, this problem in adults is just as serious and urgent an emergency as it is in kids.

Most of us can parrot the symptoms of pediatric epiglottitis easily; drooling, fever, sharp pain in the throat, stridor, the tripod position, but what does this disease look like in an adult? For the most part, it looks the same. You will find the sore throat, muffled voice, the drooling and perhaps a high fever. What's even more surprising is that this may be the first time you have heard the words "adult" and epiglottitis in the same sentence! The real problem with epiglottitis in the adult patient is the low index of suspicion. Think about it. If you transport a three-year-old with a high fever and stridor who's drooling, you expect the hospital to warm up an operating room, call anesthesia, and wake up some pediatric surgeons and ENTs. They will treat this like a real emergency. But a 20-year-old with the same presentation may not get the same response. You might just hear that the patient has a virus or a URI. In recent years there have been reports of some very tragic cases in which epiglottitis in a young adult was missed.

Management of our 24-year-old patient included transport to the hospital, where the diagnosis was made and the patient was aggressively treated and admitted. As should be observed in all suspected epiglottitis cases, the paramedics refrained from trying to visualize the throat with a tongue blade or other instrument (to keep from inducing spasm) and informed the ED of their suspicion.

So what is the issue here? For me, it simply boils down to one of education. Are we going to educate or merely train? Would any of us tolerate airline pilots who were taught the way most EMS practitioners are taught? Are we going to continue to teach a dynamic and fluid profession like EMS as if our patients were engineering problems that can afford the luxury of time and trial and error? Or will we insist that providers become comfortable with the art of assessing patients with the understanding that nothing in this business can be contained in a simple module or box? The choice is ours.

Peer Pressure

"Experience is a hard teacher because she gives the test first and the lesson later."—Vernon Law, 1960

All our lives we've been told by our mothers, fathers, teachers and coaches, "Do the right thing." In most cases, we don't need a postgraduate course in medical ethics or a Supreme Court decision to know right from wrong. And if you listen to EMS people for any length of time, you'll realize that they are obsessed with doing the right thing.

But it's not always black-and-white. Sometimes it's a matter of who we're doing the right thing for. Often, pre-hospital practitioners forge tight, collegial relationships with the police and firefighters they work with on the streets. It is also true for relationships with the ED nurses and physicians. You have to wonder, though, if these intimate working relationships create difficulties in patient care. Let's examine this case to find out.

Scenario

Your paramedic ambulance is dispatched to an MVA involving a police vehicle. The dispatcher advises you to use caution because the fire department is also en route to the scene. As you approach the scene, you see a column of smoke and several police vehicles. Fire engulfs one police car. The scene erupts in total chaos as police officers scream for you to help one of their own—a supine 30-year-old police officer whose uniform is smoldering.

As you approach him, the patient is taking labored breaths—about 24 per minute. Your quick survey shows that he has third-degree burns over 90% of his body. He's also making stridorous noises every time he takes a breath and has singed nasal hair and carbonaceous sputum. Because the patient is semiconscious, you elect to ventilate him with the bag-valve mask. You find the patient difficult to bag and decide to intubate him. You perform the laryngoscopy and find his airway swollen, red and burned with carbon as far as you can see. Your attempt at endotracheal intubation is unsuccessful. As you resume bagging him, your partner and other personnel prep the patient for transport.

As you're trying to do four things at once, the police sergeant tells you that their police helicopter is landing five blocks away to take you and the patient to the burn center in an adjacent borough. You think about this for a moment: You have a patient with an unstable airway and serious burns. The patient is also a cop, someone you've worked with—a member of the team. If there is ever a time to do the right thing, this is it.

Your training tells you that this patient needs to go to the nearest hospital, which also happens to be a trauma center, to have his airway stabilized. You know you should inform the sergeant, but you don't want to be viewed as not doing the best for a colleague. You dread the thought of this patient's airway swelling shut 1,000 feet above the city in a cramped helicopter, but you yield to the peer pressure and agree to send him by air.

You place the patient in the helicopter and the 10-minute transfer begins. His vital signs become unstable and he begins to lose consciousness. It becomes difficult to squeeze the BVM; you make another unsuccessful attempt at intubation. You are now unable to ventilate the patient. You resort to protocol and attempt a needle cricothyrotomy but due to the swelling of the tissues you are unable to get the catheter into the trachea. The patient is now in cardiorespiratory arrest.

Lessons learned
What can we take from this sorry situation? What could you have done better? Clearly, you should have followed protocol earlier and taken this patient to the nearest hospital. His airway instability should have been the most pressing issue to the EMS team. His burns did not require the immediate attention that they received. This patient was clearly too unstable to be airlifted from the scene to a burn center. Did the need to do what seemed to be the right thing by going along with peer pressure play into your decision?

When doing the right thing, remember whom you are doing it for. The choice is yours.

5
MEDICAL EMERGENCIES

Take Two Aspirin?

"Sweets grown common lose their dear delight."
—Shakespeare, Sonnet CII

As prehospital practitioners, we become comfortable with equipment, procedures and medications. We don't treat these things as dangerous implements, but rather as tools of our trade. The average person would be afraid to even handle a defibrillator. Ever watched an uninitiated person handle defibrillator paddles for the first time? It's like watching a person holding a gun for the first time: They act as if one of the paddles will jump out of their hand and bite them.

Because we handle these things every day, one wonders where the novelty goes. Familiarity breeds contempt among patients as well. Often, patients treat medicines with casual concern, and because they take the same medications at the same time every day these folks can become careless. This can result in the misuse of a common medication, producing uncommon results.

Scenario

You spend the last half of your 4 to 12 shift chauffeuring your partner, Red, to every hardware store in your response area, looking for a part he needs to fix his pool's filter pump. You listen to agonizing details of the pump breakage and endure Red's whining about it blowing on the hottest, most humid weekend of the summer. While you travel to the second of two Home Depots in your area, the dispatcher mercifully announces your next assignment: "43 X-ray, respond to an unconscious diabetic, 7106 Park Lane South off Metropolitan Ave. Time is 1510."

As you respond, you think it unsurprising that a diabetic would have problems coping in such hot, humid weather. On arrival, you find a 47-year-old, unconscious male, taking rapid, deep breaths. His rate of breathing is 43; pulse is 120. As you ensure an open airway, you smell for the fabled acetone odor to the breath and notice nothing. The patient's skin is hot and dry—not the cool, clammy skin you've seen in insulin shock patients. You consider heat stroke, but the house is air-conditioned and the room is cool.

As Red places the patient on oxygen and starts an IV, the patient's family tells you that he takes his insulin regularly and watches what he eats. They also tell you that he has taken a lot of aspirin during the past few days to ease arthritis pain in his lower back. They say that prior to his passing out, the patient vomited and complained about abdominal pain and ringing in his ears.

By this time, Red has started the IV and drawn a blood sample. You calibrate your glucometer and put in the sample, expecting a high glucose reading to confirm your impression of a patient in diabetic coma/ketoacidosis (DKA).

Although the patient has some DKA hallmarks—the rapid, deep breaths (Kussmaul's breathing), dry skin and rapid pulse—the glucometer tells you that the patient's glucose is 122, clearly not what you had expected.

As you move the patient to your ambulance, he has a seizure and becomes apneic. As you drive to the hospital, your partner intubates and bags the patient. Red tells you when the patient regains his pulse.

At the ED, you move the patient to the hospital stretcher and present the case to the doctor. She interrupts you and asks for a salicylate level to be drawn quickly. She also orders a ventilator, a gastric tube and activated charcoal followed by ipecac syrup. You're stunned because just minutes ago you were convinced that, notwithstanding the glucometer, this was probably a DKA patient who had a seizure. The blood work later confirms that this was an accidental aspirin overdose. The patient recovered.

Conclusion

Medication doesn't get any more over-the-counter (OTC) than aspirin. We take aspirin for such varied ailments as heart trouble, headache or muscle pain with as little thought as if we were taking a multivitamin. If my experience is any barometer, most of you now see more complications, such as GI bleeds, resulting from an increase in daily aspirin dosing in the past few years. Many more patients now present with toxic levels of aspirin and other OTC medications. We need to suspect OTC overdoses early in our assessments.

Fools Rush Through

"Our main business is not to see what lies at a distance, but to do what lies clearly at hand." —*Thomas Carlyle*

I wish I had a dime for every time someone approached me while I was assessing a patient and said, "Stop asking questions, and just take him to the hospital!" Sometimes our patient's problem is obvious, and the best treatment is to drive quickly to the hospital.

Everybody wants to save time. Drive down a highway in any city and you'll wonder where everyone is going in such a hurry. This problem isn't exclusive to highways, either. Recently, I read an article in the *Long Island Newsday* in which the writer, Paul Vitello, stated, "New York City Transit officials decided that in order to save time, subway conductors would drop the word 'please' when alerting passengers to stand clear of the closing doors. By trimming the word please, they said, each train would save five seconds per station stop. This would save many minutes per day."

Can we in EMS save time by talking less and doing more? Is this sometimes appropriate? This case may reveal the answer.

Scenario
The weather is great one nice summer morning, and you and your partner drive to the park to enjoy some sunshine. All is right with the world: You have a 20-oz. Starbuck's coffee and *The New York Times* at your disposal. Your partner, Ronnie, rests comfortably with a cinnamon bun in one hand and the racing form in the other.

Naturally, the dispatcher calls with an assignment to interrupt your mutual peace: "43 X-ray, respond to an unconscious female, 444 Lindsey St., corner of Rachel Blvd. Time out: 1002."

As you respond, your mind runs through the possibilities. Is this a cardiac arrest, a drug OD or one of the other countless possibilities? You pull up to find a frantic man holding a young infant in his arms. The man tells you that his wife won't wake up. You find the 28-year-old woman in bed, taking sonorous respirations that vary in rate and depth.

As you open her airway and your partner begins the assessment, the husband tells you she had a baby six days ago. She has been doing well except for some minor swelling of her legs during the past few days. The husband further reports that she has a history of diabetes. He can't tell you anything more.

The patient's BP is 188/124, and her pulse is bounding at 50. Her only response to painful stimuli: She decorticates. You and your partner recognize a critical patient. You intubate and ventilate her with 100% oxygen and make your way to your vehicle. Ronnie thinks it's probably a stroke with increased intracranial pressure and alerts the ED.

During transport you start an IV but give the patient no medications. As you place the patient on the hospital gurney and present her case to the ED physician, you finish the paperwork for the call wondering why an otherwise healthy, 28-year-old woman would have a stroke? The answer comes later when the ED doc tells you that you did a great job earlier on "that woman with eclampsia."

Confused, you ask yourself how could it be eclampsia. The patient didn't have a seizure, and she had the baby six days ago. Then the doc tells you that eclampsia can manifest itself either by a coma or seizure and can occur up to a week after delivery. The swelling of the legs and history of diabetes make up part of the picture. He also says that you took the right course by hustling her in when you weren't sure what was going on. Energized with this information, you look for Ronnie to share the important information with him.

An old mentor once told me that sometimes patients hurt themselves enough to die. Can you find that in a textbook? Nope. Going beyond the textbooks is a great and necessary thing. As I was writing this, I read the eclampsia sections in two paramedic texts, and neither text mentions that eclampsia can occur up to one week post-partum. Lesson learned by the student reading the text: Once the infant is delivered, eclampsia cannot occur.

EMS personnel need to understand that textbooks don't have enough room to present all the nuances of every illness. Experience can teach you how to fill in the blanks. But when it doesn't, it makes sense to move quickly to a medical facility where other members of the medical team can help unravel the medical mystery.

EMS Apprenticeships

*"Knowledge and timber shouldn't be much
used 'til they are seasoned."*
—Oliver Wendell Holmes

EMS personnel regard clinical experience highly because of its effectiveness as a training mechanism. Because classroom scenarios and practice can't reproduce the actual stresses and responses of real-world street medicine, a mechanism should be in place to build on the skills and thought processes learned in the classroom. Other professions call the clinical internship an apprenticeship.

Most of us accept that physicians can't learn their trade in only four years. They perform a residency for a period of time to master specific fields. Similarly, on completion of prehospital credentialing programs, most of us function at a basic competency level. That is, we can perform the basic requirements of our job without hurting patients. Because of the omnipresent learning curve, many EMS facilities/companies have implemented an internship or apprenticeship program for new hires. For good reasons, most establishments prohibit inexperienced EMTs and medics from working together for a designated length of time. This case illustrates the hazard of not having that apprenticeship.

Scenario

While working a 4 p.m.-to-midnight shift with a fellow graduate of your paramedic program, you consider how lucky both of you are. After all, you were both hired a month ago as full-time paramedics for a hospital that provides 9-1-1 coverage for the city. The two of you have looked forward to working together ever since those classroom days.

First call: the dispatcher sends you to the county jail. You arrive to find a 24-year-old male who's complained of difficulty breathing for 45 minutes. He had been arrested for becoming verbally abusive while arguing about a traffic ticket and suddenly became short of breath while in the police car. At that time, he was taken to an ED and treated. The jailer gives you the hospital chart, which indicates that the patient arrived at the hospital two hours ago in minimal distress with bilateral wheezes in his chest. He had a non-productive cough. At the time his vital signs were blood pressure 140/72, pulse 90 and respirations 20. The hospital treatment included oxygen and an infusion of aminophylline. The patient felt better, was wheezing less after treatment and was sent back to the jail.

The record also states that the patient has had asthma since childhood and takes an oral bronchodilator and an Isuprel inhaler. The patient tells you he has used the Isuprel at least five times in the last 45 minutes. Your examination reveals the patient's vital signs: blood pressure 154/82, pulse 130 and irregular and respirations 28. He's afebrile and not cyanotic. His lungs produce diffuse wheezes, and he seems to ventilate adequately. His ECG shows sinus tachycardia with occasional premature ventricular contractions (PVCs).

You and your partner discuss treatments. Your protocol allows you to administer an albuterol or metaproterenol inhaler or epinephrine up to 0.4 mg subcutaneously, under standing orders. The protocol states that you must get a physician's order if you wish to give magnesium sulfate or methylprednisolone. Your partner wants to give the patient a shot of epinephrine. After all, the patient hasn't responded well to the hospital treatment, and his inhaler hasn't helped at all. You agree with this line of treatment, having no point of reference because this is the worst asthmatic patient you have seen. You now regret having performed your ambulance clinical hours on the slowest call volume unit simply because it was the closest to home.

You draw up the 0.4 mg of 1:1,000 epinephrine and administer the subcutaneous injection. Within three minutes, the patient suffers a cardiac arrest. Despite vigorous efforts by you and the hospital staff, the patient cannot be resuscitated.

Lessons learned

Was this patient's death just bad luck for our newbie medics (and the patient)? As I see it, the major issue here is that the two people working together had paramedic cards with wet ink—a bad idea. Would an experienced medic know that the use of certain inhaled bronchodilators are associated with sudden death in asthmatics? Would they know that asthma often leads to acidosis and that giving epinephrine in the face of acidosis can lead to fatal arrhythmias? Would they realize if they use a bronchodilator then they should choose one that has the majority of effects on the lungs—not one that puts a chemical stress test on the heart?

Do you know the answer to these questions? I don't. But I do know that apprenticeship is a concept that has worked for electricians, carpenters and others for years, why not for EMS?

Sherlock Holmes, EMT

"You know everybody is ignorant,
only on different subjects."
—Will Rogers

As a medic, have you ever felt like you're in a detective
story? You know what I mean: always looking for clues;
handling suspects that refuse to answer questions truth-
fully, querying bystanders whose recall is questionable?
How about the victims who can't tell you what happened
because they either don't know or are such poor historians that they can't be relied on for an accurate appraisal
of their own experience. *Example:* a 50-year-old male
who has chest pain. When you ask him if he has a history of heart problems, he says he doesn't. But when
asked about medication, he says he's taking nitroglycerin, digoxin and lasix.

Even more memorable is the gentleman my partner
and I found seizing on the sidewalk some years ago in
Manhattan. We asked a man who identified himself as

the patient's brother if the patient was an epileptic. His answer: "Hell, no, my brother's no epileptic—he's a Baptist like me!"

Some detective stories are easier to solve than others, as we will see after examining this case.

Scenario

It's 3 a.m. You and your partner sip your second coffees of the shift. The discussion, which began with an earnest difference of opinion on whether paramedic programs should require a year of EMT experience in all applicants prior to acceptance, has degenerated into a dispute. For the hundredth time, your partner tells you, "When I was a student, I walked a hundred blocks, in blinding snow, uphill in both directions to get to class." Knowing your partner as you do, you realize it's time to nix the conversation. The dispatcher calls you for an assignment just in time: an unconscious female.

You arrive on scene to find a 40-year-old female unresponsive on the couch. Her family last saw her watching TV before 11 p.m. She never came to bed. Her only history is that she had knee surgery two weeks ago with no complications. Her family denies diabetes, heart, lung or blood pressure problems or seizure disorders. The only medication that she takes is ibuprofen 400 mg, as needed for post-op pain. She refilled the prescription yesterday.

The patient is unresponsive to verbal or painful stimuli, her BP is 102/70, pulse is 110 and regular, respirations are regular at 22/min. Her pupils are normal, equal and reactive to light. There are no signs of recreational drug use, and the family confirms this. Her skin is pale and clammy. Your partner checks for orthostatic changes or signs of abdominal rigidity. Finding none, you learn that her last period was a week ago. And she wasn't complaining of abdominal pain earlier that evening.

Your partner gives you a quizzical look which says, "What's the deal here?" We have symptoms but no obvious causes. Outstanding. We get to play Holmes and Watson in the middle of the night.

The two of you place the patient on oxygen, an ECG monitor, draw blood and start an IV. Your partner places the blood in the glucometer and whistles. The patient's blood glucose is 30. How is that possible? You give the patient a glucose bolus and thiamine as per your standing orders. She wakes up 30 seconds later and is reassuring her worried family within two minutes. You transport her to the hospital without incident. Another life saved.

Later in the week, the patient calls the station to thank you and tells you her prescription for ibuprofen was refilled with glucotrol by mistake. Glucotrol is a medication that diabetics take orally to lower their blood sugar. You and your partner take note of the pharmacy, so you don't go there to have your prescriptions filled and argue how long it will take the media to run a story on this mix-up.

Here we have a patient who is clearly sick with no obvious cause. Have you ever been faced with such a situation? Most of us have. We usually assume that the cause must be some exotic combination of unlikely events when, frequently, the cause is not exotic at all.

For example, several years ago a station wagon pulled up to our ambulance with an unconscious elderly diabetic. The family realized that she was acting strange and tried to give her the candy they regularly bought at the supermarket. Terrified that the candy had not made the lady more responsive, the family feared that she had had a stroke. Honestly, so did we—until realizing the family had given her sugarless candy.

Sometimes, you have to examine the likely suspects to solve the puzzle.

Rules to Work By

"Repetition is the branding iron of education."

Are rules useful to us? Yes. They give our existence structure. Rules and guidelines add to our safety and provide us with boundaries. Popular sentiment aside, boundaries are good things. As children, we learn that certain things are not acceptable. In adolescence, we learn that we are entitled to certain rights, but (more importantly) that others have rights as well. *A common example:* Your right to extend your fist ends where my nose begins.

In EMS, we find many of these common rules couched in clichés and platitudes that are drilled into our brains by repetition. Does "red means stop and green means go" ring a bell? Life's little rules have counterparts in our jobs, as demonstrated in this case.

Scenario
Your ambulance is dispatched to a sick adult female. You

down your cappuccino as your partner begins to weave through traffic en route to the assignment.

Several minutes later, you arrive to find a 30-year-old female, vomiting. Between heaves, she says she has had diffuse abdominal pain for the past two days. She also mentions that she has an appointment to see her private physician tomorrow morning. She reports feeling nauseated, and the pain seems to be in the lower left side of her abdomen and in her left shoulder. She has no medical history and does not wish to go to the hospital. (Her mother called 9-1-1 from another location.) Her vital signs are BP 120/78, pulse 100 and regular, respirations 14 and normal. Capillary refill is under two seconds and her skin is warm and dry. She is alert and oriented. The only medication she is currently taking is birth control pills, and she takes them exactly as prescribed. You ask the patient if it's possible she could be pregnant. She smiles wryly, and says, "No, it's not possible."

The patient again expresses her desire to go to her own doctor and not the hospital ED. While you consider this, your partner tells you he is comfortable with allowing her to refuse transport. He has seen too many system abusers this week to force this clearly ambulatory and stable patient to take the orange-and-white taxi to the emergency room. After all, isn't that what personal physicians are for?

You're uncomfortable with accepting a refusal from this patient because you recall someone at a continuing medical education session telling you that "females of childbearing age with belly pain should be assumed to have an ectopic pregnancy until the hospital proves otherwise." With that pearl in mind, you insist on taking her to the hospital for evaluation. You have learned from experience to trust that little voice of doubt that speaks up occasionally. The patient reluctantly gets into your ambulance. The transport proceeds smoothly until the ambulance pulls up at the hospital. The patient doubles over with pain. She looks pale and sweaty as you move her rapidly to the hospital stretcher.

Inside, the nurse quickly determines that the patient is tachycardic and hypotensive. As you fill out paperwork, the ED team moves her toward the operating room. Later, as you bring in your last patient of the tour, the staff tells you that the lady with the abdominal pain you brought in earlier did have an ectopic pregnancy. She's doing fine.

Just another day on the tightrope. Why do I allude to the "tightrope?" Well, if you had not remembered that little pearl or bothered to sit for that lecture, this situation may have come out differently.

Every decision, every choice made or not made may have ramifications. In patient care, there comes a time where silence or inaction is betrayal. Leaving a patient on scene often seems the path of least resistance. We convince ourselves that it is the right thing to do by telling ourselves that it's what the patient wants. Who told you that patients have better clinical judgment than you? Clearly, there are times patients must be left on scene against better judgment. But we don't have to be comfortable with that fact.

As we live our lives and nurture our careers, many of the rules that were hammered into us prevent us from making mistakes with our patients. These little bromides ensure that we don't forget the basic rules of patient care.

Hidden in Plain Sight

*"Where the telescope ends, the microscope begins.
Which of the two has the grander view?"*
—*Victor Hugo,* Les Miserables

How is EMS like a penny? Is this a credible question, or have I finally gone around the bend? Bear with me on this one. The one-cent piece is an omnipresent object, something most of us handle and use each day. You probably have one in your pocket now. But try to complete the following exercise without looking at a penny.

Whose image is on the front? Your final answer? Abraham Lincoln, of course. Now to the hard stuff: What are the inscriptions over Lincoln's head, behind and in front of his neck? Not so easy anymore, is it?

Over Lincoln's head it says, "In God We Trust." Behind him is the word "Liberty," and finally the minting date of the coin is in front of him. This little exercise is wonderful for pointing out things that are obvious, but not often noticed. So how is EMS like a penny? Let's look at this case to find out.

Scenario

On a beautiful Monday in New York, you tell your partner, Karen, about your week's vacation in Maine. You're refreshed, the fish were cooperative, and you tried your hand at kayaking—albeit with mixed results. That's when the dispatcher calls: "Medic 44x respond to a report of an elderly male with abdominal pain, 22-40 John Street off Lewis Drive. Time out is 1418." As you weave through midday traffic, you consider the assessment possibilities. The patient could have a myocardial infarction, a gastrointestinal bleed or some other life-threatening malady.

The two of you arrive on scene. An elderly man, naked and groaning in pain, answers your knock on the door. You immediately note that the patient has fecal matter smeared on him and his back is covered with bedsores. You notice other areas of the patient's skin are dry, cracking and breaking down as well.

After you glove and gown, your partner helps you wrap the patient in a bed sheet. The patient, a 77-year-old retired police officer, is conscious and alert and complains of pain in his abdomen just below the umbilicus. He also complains of nausea and vomiting. You take his vitals: BP is 92/78; heart rate 120; and respiration 28. You place the patient on high-flow oxygen and a cardiac monitor. The monitor displays sinus tachycardia at a rate of 120.

The patient's abdomen is distended. His skin turgor is poor, and his neck veins are flat in the supine position. He denies any heart history and says his only hospitalization was three years earlier for a hernia operation. When the BLS ambulance crew arrives, they ask if you'd like them to transport the patient. You think about it. The condition in which you found the patient makes it obvious he doesn't get out of bed much, not even to go to the bathroom. But he's clearly hurting bad enough to get out of bed to let you in the door. You tell the EMTs that you'll transport the patient.

You place an IV and administer a fluid challenge. The patient's vitals improve, but his pain remains unrelenting. The transport to the ED proves uneventful.

Outcome
A week later the ED physician who admitted the patient tells you the elderly gentleman was diagnosed with a small bowel obstruction that probably stemmed from his earlier hernia operation. He says this is not unusual because abdominal surgery is notorious for causing loops of the small bowel to stick together (adhesions) so often that prior abdominal surgery is implicated in up to 60% of such obstructions. In your patient's case, the obstruction was strangulated, causing the bowel section to become necrotic. Untreated, a strangulated obstruction carries a 100% mortality rate. However, if treated within 36 hours, mortality decreases to 8%. The patient recovers from surgery and survives.

When we're new to EMS, our senses are hyper-acute. We can vividly recall every aspect of a case. You can probably remember the first patient you ever treated, your first cardiac arrest, etc. You may remember certain odors and other less obvious things and can relate the episode as if it happened yesterday. After we've been in the field for a while, we tend to think we've seen everything at least once and can become complacent. But by doing so, we can miss or discount history, presentation, even symptoms. Remember to examine the entire patient before making treatment or transport decisions.

Masquerade

"Things are seldom as they seem; skim milk masquerades as cream."—Sir William Schwenk Gilbert

I've been to my share of parties in my time, but they were always run of the mill—birthdays, holidays, the good-luck-on-the-new-job or sorry-that-you're-retiring party. I always hoped that a masquerade party would come along. Not only would it give me a chance to demonstrate my moulage techniques, but also enjoy watching folks trying to be somebody or something that they're not.

You can meet some interesting people at such masked parties: Napoleon, pirates, Caesar, Al Gore, etc. You can also occupy your time trying to decide who's behind the mask or makeup. You see the mask; you don't see the real content. What does this have in common with EMS? Read this case to find out.

Scenario

You and your partner, Eric, stop for lunch at a Chinese restaurant. You just get the food to the table when the dispatcher calls and assigns you to "an unconscious overdose, 43-10 Frank Street, corner of Sperl Ave. Time out 1323."

"That's Rudy's address again," you exclaim. Rudy is your personal nemesis, a heroin addict who always seems to drop when you're on duty. Two weeks ago you were on duty when he overdosed on Valium, sleeping pills and codeine. Then he took a heroin hit and followed this brew with a pint of gin. During your radio conversation with the medical control physician, he asked what you wanted to do with the patient. You thought about replying, "Shake him up and pour him over ice." Rudy overdoses regularly, and a smidgen of naloxone has proven his salvation many times before. Now this miscreant is unconscious again.

As you pull up at the address this time, Rudy's roommate directs you inside, telling you that your patient had staggered around the room and vomited before he passed out. You find Rudy supine and comatose, his airway open and maintainable with position. He's breathing at a rate of 12 per minute. The respirations are grossly irregular in depth. Lung sounds are normal. Pulse is bounding at 100, and his blood pressure is 190/110. The patient's pupils are pinpoint and nonreactive to light. His skin feels warm to your touch.

As you place the patient on high-flow oxygen, your partner tries to obtain IV access. He has difficulty finding a viable vein, but succeeds on his third attempt. You draw blood and run the saline IV at KVO. Your standing orders in such cases are to draw blood, establish vascular access and administer 25 gm of dextrose to reverse hypoglycemia. The next intervention is thiamine (vitamin B1), an essential ingredient to enable the brain to use the sugar. You're supposed to administer the thiamine as an IV bolus of 100 mg through the IV set.

In addition to these therapies, protocol dictates the use of naloxone at 2 mg IV bolus to reverse the effects of opiates in suspected overdoses. The protocol allows you to administer the naloxone first if you strongly suspect a narcotic OD. Your partner administers the naloxone. You wait several minutes for it to work, then administer the dextrose and thiamine. None of the medications appear to have a positive impact on the patient's condition. Based on your perfunctory assessment of the patient's vital signs and pupils—and little else—you feel that a second bolus of 2 mg naloxone is indicated.

You administer the second dose of naloxone with no response. Your protocol allows you to administer a total of five 2-mg boluses of naloxone. Although you recall that Rudy has never required more than two rounds of naloxone to completely destroy his $100 high, you proceed with the full protocol allowance.

Several minutes later, without fanfare, Rudy stops breathing and loses his pulse. You begin a futile resuscitation attempt and transport him to the hospital, just four blocks away.

Not just another overdose
A week later your medical director calls you and Eric into her office. She informs you that Rudy died as a result of a pontine hemorrhage. Deep in the brain, the pons is an area of nerve tissue that controls the inspiratory phase of respiration. Symptoms of a pontine hemorrhage include stagger, nausea and vomiting, high

temperature and pinpoint pupils.

Although the medical director understands why you initially treated the patient as a narcotic OD, she cannot countenance the fact that you continued administering a drug that was clearly not working and delayed quick transport to the nearby hospital. She tells you that you'll be informed of her decision. You both leave her office wondering if you'll ever be allowed to treat a patient again.

Pit-bull effect

This case demonstrates the pit-bull effect—holding on to a preconceived notion and not letting go, no matter what the facts are. In social contexts it's called bias and is every bit as unpalatable in that venue as in EMS. A masquerade costume can effectively disguise the person beneath, but you shouldn't endanger the lives of your patients by allowing bias to interfere with your assessment and treatment decisions.

Take a Second Look at Your First Impression

"When you have eliminated the impossible, whatever remains, however improbable, must be the truth."
—*Sir Arthur Conan Doyle,* The Sign of Four

You get only one chance to make a good first impression. If your parents raised you like mine did me, you've probably heard that platitude your entire life. Whether going to a job interview or meeting your date's family for the first time, you heard that first impressions count.

Unfortunately, appearance issues sometimes obscure matters of substance. EMS providers fall prey to this phenomenon too. We pride ourselves on our ability to ferret out a patient's diagnosis based on our impressions. But do these impressions always lead us to the correct answer? Let's examine this case to find out.

Scenario
One spring evening you pull up to a Chinese restaurant to grab dinner with your partner. Before you have time

to place your order, the dispatcher summons you for a "38-year-old female, sick at a wedding reception; Marino's Catering Hall, 43-10 Shearman Ave., corner of Mark Place. Time out is 1934." A sick call at a caterer's banquet hall. The bride probably got cold feet.

As you drive toward the location, your mind drifts back to the day you got married. As you took the long walk down the aisle, you felt petrified. You can easily see how someone can get physically sick when they get that nervous. You pull up on scene, and someone directs you to a small room where you find the patient—not the bride, but one of the bridesmaids.

You interview the patient, who complains of feeling nauseated. She says she vomited several times during the past 30 minutes. She has no relevant medical history—except for an ear infection (she saw the doctor for it yesterday). She usually takes only birth control pills, but earlier today took two Keflex pills prescribed for her ear infection. She claims to have eaten only salad. She denies being pregnant and tells you her period ended yesterday.

As your partner obtains the patient's vital signs, the patient begins to sneeze and cough vigorously. "Great," you think, "Now I'm gonna get an ear infection or pneumonia."

The patient's nose begins to run and she says she has trouble breathing. You administer oxygen. Vitals are pulse 110, blood pressure 88/50, respiration 20 and labored. You auscultate her lungs and hear wheezing. You think to yourself, "There's no way that nasty bacteria moved from her ear to her chest overnight."

The patient then tells you her skin feels itchy and warm. During your examination you notice some raised blotches on her skin. Your thoughts turn immediately to anaphylaxis and rapid transport. You place the patient quickly on the stretcher and get her in the ambulance. Although she has no history of anaphylaxis and doesn't report intake of penicillin, peanuts, shellfish or any other usual suspect, her condition fits the symptomology.

Your partner starts two, large-bore IVs. You call medical control and receive orders for subcutaneous epinephrine and IV diphenhydramine. Your partner administers the medications, and the patient's condition and vital signs improve prior to arrival at the hospital. You transfer care to the ED staff and go back in service.

After the call
You return to the ED two hours later, and the ED doctor fills you in. The patient had an anaphylactic reaction to the Keflex. Patients commonly have anaphylactic reactions the first time they take a medication. This patient had a delayed response because she took the drug orally. The physician says injected drugs act much faster and also tells you abdominal complaints are common.

The patient has an uneventful recovery. Even though you feel as if you zeroed in on the patient's problem a little slowly, the doctor says you and your partner did well by treating the patient as aggressively as you did.

First impressions can prove truly lasting ones, sometimes to the peril of those involved. The reception of a sick call can sometimes mislead us. In this case, the atmosphere of the catering hall and wedding all conspired to influence the providers' judgment in a certain direction. The ability to filter interference on a dynamic scene remains perhaps the greatest asset prehospital providers can have. No one can teach this to us; it's an art developed in the heat of battle.

Awkward Assessments

"Man is the only animal that blushes. Or needs to."
—*Mark Twain*

"Yes," the talk show host insisted, "Women and men are different." Wow. After 13 years of marriage, that didn't come as a great revelation to me. You could also say children and adults differ: Children are small, brutally honest little folks who say what's on their mind without pretense and will candidly answer any questions about their bodies or health. Adults, on the other hand, are more self-conscious.

As a rule, female adult patients I've interviewed over the years tend to honestly describe symptoms without spinning the history or exam. Women tend to give honest answers—even for an embarrassing problem.

But I've noticed that men hate giving embarrassing information—even to their physicians. In fact, until former presidential candidate Bob Dole admitted on national television that he had erectile dysfunction, men wouldn't talk with their doctors about it. Can fear of embarrassment create problems in the prehospital environment? Let's examine this case to find out.

Scenario
One summer evening you're working with your partner on an ALS ambulance. It's a nice night in the big city—low humidity and quiet enough to enjoy the sights and sounds. Dispatch shakes you from your reverie: "Medic 43X, respond for an adult male complaining of severe back pain, 1445 William Drive, off O'Connor Ave. Time out is 2002."

As your partner drives to the scene, you wonder out loud where the BLS units are and why you're getting their assignment. On scene, you find Larry Zach, a 33-year-old police officer. Between paroxysms of pain, he tells you he was lifting a heavy object into his police car and suddenly experienced severe back pain. He says he's felt this way for about seven hours, has vomited and has severe nausea. His wife says he's been sweating profusely since he came home, but he doesn't have a fever.

His vital signs: Blood pressure 146/88, pulse 110 and respirations 28. You administer oxygen via non-rebreather mask, initiate cardiac monitoring and establish an IV of normal saline. The patient's ECG reveals sinus tachycardia at a rate of 110.

When you ask about the intensity of his problem, Zach tells you he's never felt worse pain, and it's unrelieved by position or rest. He then asks his wife to leave the room. When she leaves, he tells you the pain is moving from his back to his scrotum. He says he was too embarrassed to mention it before.

You pull on your gloves and examine his scrotum, finding it swollen and tender to the touch. You place the patient on your stairchair and gently apply ice packs around his scrotum in an attempt to ease his pain. During transport, the patient admits he should have called earlier to report the problem. Because of his embarrassment and because he didn't want anyone touching his private parts, he tolerated the pain as long as possible.

At the hospital, physicians place a doppler on the scrotum and confirm there's no blood supply to the swollen testicle. They hustle the victim into surgery, but they can't save the testicle.

Testicular torsion
The next week your medical director conducts a continuing medical education class for your department, and Zach's case comes up. The doctor informs you that testicular torsion is a legitimate emergency caused by the testicle twisting on the spermatic cord, interrupting its blood supply. It can be caused by trauma or occur spontaneously.

Testicular torsion most often occurs at age one or during puberty, but any male between the ages of five months and 41 years old is at risk. *The presentation:* sudden and unrelenting scrotal pain that often radiates to the back, accompanied by swelling, nausea and vomiting.

The patient must be treated with cold application and rapid transport in the first two to six hours after torsion occurs to prevent tissue death and have any hope of salvaging the testicle. Other conditions suggested by this presentation include kidney stones, epididymitis or musculoskeletal pain.

Discussion
We've all seen patients in obvious discomfort trying to be stoic. Myocardial infarction patients are famous for

this. I've found countless chest-pain patients taking multiple stomach meds or topical pain relievers when they should have called 9-1-1. This case is no different.

Patients with testicular pain are almost always embarrassed and may insist the pain is in their back. In this case, embarrassment cost the patient dearly. Please remember it's our job to ask tough questions and insist on honest, complete answers.

Distracted by the Facts

"The eye altering, alters all."
—William Black, The Mental Traveler

While driving home recently, I noticed the warning inscribed on my right-side rearview mirror. It warns, "Objects in mirror are closer than they appear." I find it amazing that a simple change in perception can distort things so dramatically. Seeing hazards in the correct perspective can obviously make all the difference in the world when we perform important tasks like driving an ambulance or flying an airplane. It's also important when we assess our patients. For an example, let's examine this case.

Scenario
You're getting the day's first cup of coffee when the dispatcher tones you out. "Elderly male, unknown condition, at the Saldin Institute, 324 Brian Road, at the corner of Kelly Ave. Time out is 0650." You know Saldin is a large facility that provides care for geriatric patients and

houses a psychiatric wing as well.

On arrival, you're directed to the bedside of a 78-year-old male. The staff tells you he's suffering new-onset tremors, continuing drowsiness and has had a fever of 102° for the past 24 hours. They also tell you he's been irritable lately. His only worrisome history is high blood pressure and the fever. *His vital signs:* blood pressure 134/84, pulse 80, respirations 18. A staff nurse tells you he takes a beta-blocker for the blood pressure and has received an antibiotic for the fever.

As your partner administers oxygen, you connect the ECG. It shows a heart rate of 80 with no ectopy. The 12-lead reveals no abnormality. You mentally start to pigeonhole the patient into a non-critical category.

Not to miss anything, you assess him for neck stiffness to rule out meningitis. He can move his head freely. You listen to his chest and hear rhonchi and other low-pitched rumbles on his right side. The staff now informs you the in-house physician, who treated the patient earlier that morning, had expressed concern about right-side pneumonia. You note the patient also has a non-productive cough, reinforcing your belief in the doctor's pneumonia suspicion. While working on the patient, you again notice how warm he is. You start an IV of normal saline.

The staff tells you his doctor is waiting for him at North Area Hospital. It's 15 minutes away, but your patient seems stable, so you decide to transport him to where his doctor awaits.

During transport, the patient becomes less responsive and seems intoxicated. *His current vitals:* blood pressure 126/78, pulse 90, respirations 20. Solid, stable vitals—nothing requiring advanced therapies, you believe.

On arrival at the ED, you present the patient to the triage nurse, who sends the patient directly to a bed. The patient's physician begins her evaluation while you complete your paperwork and get a signature. You get back on the road and notify dispatch you're back in service.

Discussion
Several days later your medical director calls you in to explain your thoughts and actions on the Saldin call. You recount the dispatch and patient condition when you arrived. It seemed as if the patient had an infection, probably pneumonia, and you hydrated him via IV and transported him to the hospital. Your medical director agrees the diagnosis was pneumonia.

The problem: Your patient's doctor called. The ED checked the patient's blood glucose because he was minimally responsive on arrival and found the patient had a blood glucose level of 18—clearly a medical emergency. You failed to conduct a complete assessment, and—because of it—the patient suffered severe brain damage due to hypoglycemia. He probably won't survive.

You should've remembered from your training that a fever increases metabolic rate and can cause profound hypoglycemia. The patient was on a beta-blocker, putting him at further risk. The beta-blocker masked the tachycardia that accompanies hypoglycemia. Your director asks why you didn't obtain a blood glucose reading in a less-than-alert patient. You can offer no answer.

Conclusion
In this case, the providers bought into the doctor's presumptive diagnosis of pneumonia. They concentrated solely on treating that problem, ignoring changes in the patient's condition that warranted more immediate care.

You know your protocols call for a blood glucose check on patients who aren't alert. The object in the mirror (the hypoglycemic condition) was closer to you than it appeared. You should have recognized the indications for checking the patient's blood glucose reading. The pneumonia posed the more distant threat. We need to keep our minds open to all possibilities, no matter how remote they may seem.

Diagnostic Pearls

"If the blind lead the blind, both shall fall into the ditch."
—*Matthew 15:14*

We are all products of our training. In many cases, if our instruction was weak, major holes in our knowledge base exist. *Example:* Instructors still recommend looking for cherry red skin in cases of carbon monoxide poisoning. In the field, however, you hardly ever see this sign. Most of the time, cyanosis is evident in these cases. In fact, the only time I've ever seen cherry red skin in CO poisonings was on a corpse.

Some of the most important information an instructor can convey to students is in the form of diagnostic pearls: little maxims you can use to remember critical stuff. *Example:* Assume abdominal pain in a woman of childbearing years denotes an ectopic pregnancy until proven otherwise. Remembering this pearl could save a young woman's life. For a more in-depth example, read this case.

Scenario

You and your partner are dispatched to a diabetic emergency at 636 Brooklyn Ave. at the corner of Hawthorn Street. On scene, you find an unconscious 49-year-old male, breathing deeply at 30 times per minute. His airway remains open and maintainable with position. His skin feels warm and dry. His mouth and mucous membranes appear dry. His heart rate is 100 with a blood pressure of 120/80. Your partner places the patient on high-flow oxygen and records an ECG while you obtain the patient's history from the family.

They report he's an insulin-dependent diabetic who rarely takes his medications. He's been vomiting for the past two days and has complained of nausea and excessive thirst. The family denies the patient has any history of heart disease, respiratory problems, seizure history or allergies and says the patient doesn't smoke.

Based on what you see and hear, you believe the patient displays all the hallmarks of diabetic ketoacidosis (DKA), including increased respiratory rate. Your partner starts an IV, and you examine the patient and review the possible causes of DKA: too low an insulin dose, failure to take insulin, infection, increased stress, increased dietary intake and decreased metabolic rate.

While you continue to think, your partner reveals the glucometer won't calibrate, making it impossible to obtain a blood glucose reading. You think to yourself that giving this guy a bolus of dextrose should pose no problems, especially because his blood glucose remains unavailable. After all, instructors have drilled into your mind that all unconscious diabetics should receive dextrose because it's potentially lifesaving. Besides, bringing unconscious diabetics into the ED with single-digit glucose levels can be a real showstopper.

You continue your assessment. Something about this patient presentation isn't right. Some signs keep pulling you away from DKA. Those same instructors who hammered on you about giving dextrose to unconscious diabetics also told you that patients with DKA are seldom this deeply comatose. You remember that head trauma, drug overdose and stroke can all cause coma. These may also cause the alteration in respiratory pattern that you documented.

You secure the patient's airway and place an oropharyngeal airway. He doesn't struggle as you intubate him. While taping the tube, you notice his pupils appear unequal in size. "It sure looks like a stroke now," you think.

Per protocol, you administer naloxone to rule out opiate overdose. You don't give the patient any dextrose because you know it may exacerbate cerebral damage in stroke victims. You promptly transport the patient to the hospital, and a subsequent CT scan confirms stroke.

Discussion
Your medical director affirms that your decision not to administer dextrose was right on target. He also reaffirms your suspicions that DKA patients are almost always rousable and can typically answer questions.

Conclusion
Education in EMS and most medical fields is an interesting animal. We try to teach skills that normally can only be learned through experience. We give our students countless clues and presenting symptoms so they can recall any one of them on demand. Instructors and students must remain aware that some of these clues

may prove false. We expect them to be present in many cases, and our suspicions are aroused when they're not. As instructors, we need to teach our students to think and process patient information—not simply recall facts from memory.

6
GERIATRIC EMERGENCIES

Assessment & Specialized Pathology of the Elderly Patient

"Paramedic 43 respond to an elderly female complaining of shortness of breath and chest pain, the AnnaMaria Nursing center, 125 Fresh Pond Road, time 0403."

On arrival, you find a 78-year-old female who had complained of elbow pain for two hours. The nursing home staff reports that the patient always complains of elbow pain because of her arthritis.

The patient has a history of diabetes, chronic obstructive pulmonary disease (COPD) and arthritis, and she denies pain radiation, shortness of breath or nausea. She says that although she gets this arthritis pain frequently, it feels different this time. Because she can't elaborate further, you have to make the distinction between arthritis or an atypical myocardial infarction (MI) presentation.

Sound familiar? Geriatric calls, those involving patients over age 65, have become de rigeur in virtually all EMS venues. Because the elderly constitute the fastest growing section of the population, you'll find yourself on these calls more than ever.

Why does aging make us more likely to need EMS? After age 30, our bodies undergo significant changes. By age 60 those changes manifest themselves in our respiratory, renal, cardiovascular, nervous and musculoskeletal systems. Let's examine these and other changes in the geriatric population.

Respiratory system changes

By age 75, the vital capacity of the lungs—the amount of air they can move with maximum inhalation and maximum exhalation—may be reduced by up to 50%. In addition, the amount of oxygen carried by the arteries lowers drastically. *Example:* A normal 30-year-old has a partial pressure of oxygen (PaO_2) in their arterial blood of 90 millimeters of mercury (mm/hg); an average 70-year-old has a PaO_2 of 70 mm/hg. Clinically speaking, this reduction means that geriatric patients can't compensate well for hypoxia.

As a body ages, the respiratory tract gradually loses the hair-like projections called cilia, which—when irritated—cause us to cough and sneeze. Because of this, older people also lose their coughing and sneezing reflexes, which keep out nasty things that infect the lungs. Moist, dark and warm, the lungs constitute an ideal home for bacteria to grow, and the lungs of today's active geriatrics are routinely exposed to the outside environment. It's no surprise that older people are increasingly prone to pneumonia.

Cardiovascular system changes

Providers should remain alert to changes in older patients' cardiovascular systems. Why? Elderly patients have a profound reduction in their ability to increase their heart rates. First, with aging comes a diminished response by the body to the hormones that increase heart rate and cause blood vessel vasoconstriction. Also, the heart's specialized tissues, which carry electrical impulses, tend to work more slowly in aged patients. If this weren't enough, cardiac output drops by 30% between ages 30 and 80.

If geriatric patients can't raise their heart rates, what happens when they become injured and hypovolemic? Do they demonstrate the universal hypovolemia symptom—tachycardia? Probably not. (This doesn't even factor in elderly people who take medications to further reduce their heart rate.) All this means that providers can't count on tachycardia, a common parameter of shock, in older patients.

In addition, many geriatric patients have high blood pressure (BP). A BP of 112/70 wouldn't classify a young person as "hypotensive"; however, that BP would clearly be too low for a person whose normal BP is 160/90.

Renal system changes

Aging also affects the renal system. Total renal perfusion (blood filtered by the kidney) falls by as much as 50% in geriatric patients. In addition, by age 80, kidney weight has reduced by as much as 30–40%. The kidney shrinks with age, losing the structures that filter toxins or drugs from the blood. This process increases the amount of waste products in the blood and increases the body's intolerance to excess fluid in the bloodstream.

As renal system function declines, the chances of renal failure due to infections (e.g., pneumonia and meningitis) steadily increase. More waste and fluid in the bloodstream also negatively affect the liver, which makes elderly patients more susceptible to toxic or negative effects from medication than a younger person. This presents a reason not to fluid-load geriatric trauma patients.

Nervous system changes

Once upon a time, declining mental function was considered a byproduct of senility. But now we know this isn't necessarily true. Medications such as antihypertensives or those for pain can have profound effects, such as confusion, sleepiness or personality changes, on geriatric mental function.

Organically, by age 70, brain mass has reduced by 10%. Reduced neurotransmitters and blood flow contribute greatly to the effects of aging on the brain (e.g., decrease in the velocity of nerve conduction, changes in motor responses, changes in visual acuity, etc.). Finally, nerve impulse conduction to and from the brain slows considerably as a person ages, which directly affects the geriatric person's ability to walk, hear and see.

Musculoskeletal system changes

EMS practitioners have to remain keenly aware of the devastating effects of falls on the elderly population. Falls result in the death of almost 10,000 older adults in the United States annually. Of elderly patients hospitalized as a result of falling, 50% die within 12 months due to pulmonary emboli caused by not moving around enough, complications from bed sores, pneumonia resulting from prolonged bed rest and more. This is a frightening statistic.

Major musculoskeletal changes are associated with a person's tendency to fall. As we age, significant muscle atrophy and bone weakness (due to calcium loss) lend themselves to long-bone fractures. Many patients who appear to have fractured a hip as a result of a fall may actually have first fractured the hip due to stress on diseased bone, which caused the fall.

Additionally, many geriatric patients have thinning disks in the spine and a hunchback posture, which may result in the loss of up to 3 inches of height. Therefore, changes in their center of gravity and gait make it easier for them to fall and become injured.

Other consequences for geriatrics
- *Vision*: In my 20s, I had perfect 20/15 vision. That changed five years ago when I turned 37. First came reading glasses; now I use bifocals and prescription sunglasses. Goodbye, forever, Mr. Ray-Ban. Worsening vision remains a hallmark of aging. It creates specific problems: falls, motor vehicle accidents, accidental overdoses.
- *Thermal regulation*: The elderly are more prone to hypothermia and heat stroke than younger folks because they can't vasoconstrict peripheral vessels; they have poor circulation or other medical problems or suffer the consequences of poor nutrition. That's why we frequently find an elderly patient in a sweater or multiple layers of clothing in an apartment that's 88 degrees with the windows painted shut. With this in mind, it doesn't take a PhD in thermodynamics to figure out that heat and cold emergencies are common geriatric issues.
- *Medications*: As a person ages, their muscle mass decreases and their fat stores increase. The effect of this is not just aesthetic: Certain fat-soluble medications require that dosages be precisely individualized. Elderly patients are, therefore, more likely to build toxic levels of medications in their systems

than younger people.

- *Nutrition:* Several years ago, much was made of reports that many elderly people were malnourished—subsisting on dog food and other unusual dietary delights. The basic problem remains that—for several reasons—many people older than 65 don't have adequate food or vitamin intake to maintain health. Why?

  1. Some lack the funds to purchase high-quality, fresh, non-processed food (checked the price of fresh vegetables lately?).
  2. Loneliness and depression following the death of a spouse or contemporary cause a loss of appetite.
  3. Poorly fitting false teeth can make eating non-processed foods nearly impossible. Because vegetables, fruit and meats require adequate chewing to obtain proper nourishment, those with poorly fitting dentures or no teeth often have no nutritional recourse.
  4. As people age, they may lose their ability to taste food—as well as their appetite. Plus, gastric motility decreases, which means that food takes longer to make the trip through the gastrointestinal tract. This results in bloating, gas and constipation, which causes some geriatric people to refrain from eating.

Assessment tips

1. Communicate respectfully and openly: If a patient wears several layers of clothing, let them know that you have to remove them in order to conduct your physical assessment effectively. Keep them as informed as possible about what you're doing and

why. Once you gain their trust, they will generally comply with all your requests. *EMS tip:* Always introduce yourself; ask the patient's name and remember it. Don't call them "Honey" or "Pop." Address them by name (e.g., Mr. Smith). Speak slowly and carefully, make eye contact and be a good listener.

2. Determine chronic vs. acute illness: Elderly folks can have several illnesses at the same time. It's not unusual to have a patient with hypertension coexisting with heart disease, diabetes and COPD. When this patient complains of difficulty breathing, it requires Solomon-like wisdom to ferret out the source of the problem.

Are the crackles/rales you hear in the patient's chest due to heart failure or have they been present for months because the patient is confined to bed? Is the patient's skin turgor poor because of dehydration, or is it the result of normal skin aging? Such chronic conditions conspire to make assessment perplexing.

EMS tip: If a caregiver or family member is present, ask them, "Is this the way the patient usually looks?"

EMS tip: Check the medicine cabinet for new prescriptions. Or, if your community has a "vial of life" or similar program (whereby patients have been instructed to store all medications in the refrigerator), go to the kitchen for a look-see because these medications provide important clues in a geriatric patient history.

3. Evaluate pain perception: As we age, our response to pain diminishes, which complicates the assessment of heart and abdominal problems in particular. If an

older patient thinks they're having arthritis pain, the patient and the EMS provider may underestimate the severity of the problem.

4. Remain sensitive: Most elderly patients are concerned with the loss of autonomy. Being in a hospital is not a pleasant experience for those who take great pride in self-sufficiency; they may not report symptoms completely or accurately to avoid a trip to the ED and the accompanying bills that stress their fixed incomes.

Sometimes, a patient's underestimation of the problem or refusal of treatment and/or hospitalization may come down to a genuine fear of death.

EMS tip: Be up front with your patients. Address their fears and reassure them that you are recommending treatment or transfer in their best interest.

EMS tip: Use treatment devices that correspond to your patient's size, not age. Examples of this include blood pressure cuffs, cervical collars, etc.

Conclusion

The ever-increasing life expectancy of Americans has brought with it some interesting problems. In the past, retirement wasn't a problem because people just didn't live long enough to retire. But as people live longer, EMS can expect to see more elderly patients in the field—with more comprehensive medical histories that require exploration and treatment.

When Seniors Suffer

Your ambulance is dispatched to a call for an unconscious elderly patient. On arrival, you're met by a woman who says her mother isn't responding. As she speaks, you notice the distinct odor of beer on the daughter's breath. Inside, you find a semi-conscious 80-year-old woman, obviously malnourished, with prominent bruises in various healing stages. The patient has blood coming out her nose and mouth, snoring respirations of only 10 per minute and a blood pressure of 80/60. The daughter says her mother has fallen several times during the past two weeks, but she has no idea how the blood got in her mother's mouth. You quickly begin to suction and intubate the patient, start an IV of normal saline, package the patient and begin transport to the trauma center.

You find out later the patient is brain dead from her injuries and remains in a vegetative state for a week before she dies. When questioned by police, the daughter admits to hitting her mother, because "She kept me awake with her constant moaning." The daughter was arrested and awaits trial.

Population shift

Advances in medical care and technology, in conjunction with a decline in birthrate, have caused a profound shift in the age distribution of the U.S. population. In 1983, the U.S. Census Bureau reported 26.5 million people older than age 65 (11% of the population). Ten years later, the census indicated that 30 million people (15% of the population) in the United States were older than age 65. Experts estimate by the year 2050 approximately 49 million (20% of the population) will be older than 65.[1] With this rapid growth in the elderly population, several public blind spots regarding elderly care have developed.

Out in the open

In the past 20 years, the scourge of domestic violence and abuse has emerged from the shadows. So much so that an unsophisticated observer might have thought domestic abuse was a new problem. In reality, however, it has been a problem for years. Many of us have developed such a heightened awareness of abuse that we become naturally suspicious when an injured child or woman shows up in an ED.

Unfortunately, our suspicions don't naturally kick in when the elderly are concerned. The public doesn't recognize that many of our oldest and most vulnerable citizens are exposed to significant abuse and neglect on a daily basis.

This article defines elder abuse and describes its incidence, abuse patterns and the likely victims and abusers. It also discusses possible causes of and methods to eradicate this problem.

Definition & incidence

Elder abuse is the infliction of physical pain, injury, debilitating mental anguish, unreasonable confinement or willful deprivation of services necessary to maintain the mental and physical health of an elderly patient.[2] Nationally, the problem has reached epidemic proportions, affecting one in 25 older persons.[3] This means it's only slightly less common than child abuse.

A 1998 study contends elder abuse remains severely under-reported, estimating that a half million individuals in domestic settings were abused and/or neglected during 1996. The study indicates that for every reported incident of elder abuse or neglect, approximately five go unreported.[4] In 1996, the best national estimate was that 449,924 persons age 60 or older experienced abuse and neglect in domestic settings.[5] Of these, only 16% (70,942) were reported to and substantiated by authorities.

Identifying elder abuse

Elder abuse is often more difficult to identify than child abuse. Frequently, the elderly are socially isolated and have few interactions with people aside from their family or caregivers. In contrast, children never live alone and must attend school between ages five and 16.[6]

Look for several abuse patterns and potential indicators during your assessment of elderly patients. Physical abuse can include kicking, punching, slapping, physically restraining or raping victims. Indications include:

- Overt physical trauma;
- Restraint trauma;
- Repeated injury patterns;
- Unexplained injuries;
- Inconsistent injury explanations;
- Injuries a caregiver didn't disclose;

- Visits to several doctors or emergency departments; and
- Lags between when the injury occurred and treatment is sought.

Passive or active neglect: The caregiver fails to meet the person's physical, social or emotional needs. The factor that determines passive or active neglect is the caregiver's intent. A person actively neglecting an elderly person intentionally fails to meet their obligations.

With passive neglect, the failure is unintentional, often resulting from lack of information. Indications of passive neglect include:

- Lack of attention to personal care;
- Signs of malnourishment;
- Chronic physical or mental health problems;
- Dehydration; and
- Bed sores.

Psychological abuse: The intentional infliction of mental harm or psychological distress, ranging from insults and verbal abuse to threats of physical violence or isolation. Indications can include:

- *Psychological signs:* deference, passivity, anxiety, depression, confusion, disorientation; and
- *Behavioral signs:* lack of eye contact, evasiveness, agitation, hypervigilance, trembling.

Characteristics of the victim and the abuser: Statistically, the victim of elder abuse is a woman, age 75 or older. She's a widow with one or more chronic medical problems and physically and financially dependent on a caregiver or government entitlements.

In residence, the abuser is usually the victim's daughter. (Men don't take in their parents as often as women.) The abuser is usually unhappy with her role as a caregiver. She may be an alcoholic or have a drug problem. She may have a psychiatric history or some familial crisis may have set off a pattern of abuse. Recent investigations suggest that elder abuse is associated more with the abuser's underlying personality issues than with the stress of caring for a sick, dependent person. Many abusers were abused as children.

Possible causes of elder abuse

Elder abuse is a complex issue. There's seldom a single cause of elder abuse. Often, it stems from a complex crescendo of events. *Among the possibilities:*

Caregiver stress: Taking care of an elderly relative with multiple medical difficulties is emotionally and financially draining on caregivers and their families. Although often well-meaning, caregivers who lack the resources, skills and requisite education to care for a physically or mentally impaired older adult can experience a tremendous amount of stress. This "caregiver overload" can result in neglect or abuse.

The dependent or impaired older person: Some experts argue that as the dependency of the older adult increases, the stress and resentment of the caregiver increases.[7] Studies indicate that individuals in poor health will more likely suffer abuse than their contemporaries in good health. Caregivers who are financially dependent on the older person will more likely perpetrate abuse than financially independent caregivers. Authorities theorize that the abuse counteracts feelings of powerlessness the caregiver may experience.

External stresses: Such caregiver issues as financial problems, job stress and additional family stresses can increase the risk of elder abuse. Alcoholism, drug abuse and emotional problems can also contribute to increased risk (this correlation has been confirmed in spousal and child abuse studies).

Social isolation: In the first part of the 20th century, extended families lived in communal fashion, in enclaves surrounded by their close relatives. This created a safety net that protected the welfare of individuals within the community. We see this same phenomenon in many cloistered groups (e.g., the Amish). As the American society shifts from a communal pattern, many people are left with feelings of isolation and loneliness. Abuse patterns (elder, spousal and child) often occur in these isolated families. (Remember, isolation can indicate abuse and serve as a risk factor.)

Interfamilial violence: Individuals abused as children are predisposed to abuse others. In these families, violence is a learned behavior and a typical response to feelings of anger, hostility or lack of fulfillment. If an older person now receiving care abused their child and that child is now in the position of caregiver, they may return the abuse. Think about this cycle of violence as the "what goes around, comes around" theory.

Elder abuse checklist

Recognition—Does the patient:

  Have unexplained injuries?

  Offer inconsistent explanations of injuries?

  Show signs of restraint trauma?

  Have several injuries in various stages of healing?

  Show signs of malnourishment?

  Have bed sores?

Report your suspicions:

  Do not confront the alleged abuser.

  Report your suspicions to the police and

  ED staff. Elder abuse is against the law.

Material/financial abuse

In the assessment or treatment of the elderly, EMS personnel often hear comments from friends, neighbors or relatives that may become clues to elder abuse. These clues may be related to material or financial abuse of the victim and involve the misuse, misappropriation or exploitation of the money, property or possessions of an older person. Indications include:

- Unusual banking activity; Bank statements that no longer come to the elderly person;
- Elderly living under conditions not commensurate with the size of their estate;
- Missing belongings; Signatures on checks and documents that don't match;
- Inappropriate caregiver concerns (financial only); and New acquaintances who isolate the elderly individual from family and friends.

Prevention

Older adults should make every effort to maintain social ties with both friends and family—even if they move. The buddy system has never been more appropriate. Friends should visit the elderly in their homes, remaining vigilant for abuse signs. The elderly should participate in community affairs as much as possible and obtain legal advice for power-of-attorney, protection of assets and other important issues. Example: They should arrange for their Social Security and pension checks to be deposited directly into their bank accounts.

Allowing an elderly person to live with a person who has a substance abuse problem or a history of violent behavior is fraught with danger. If found in this environment, an older adult should be relocated to a safer environment.

Families should seek resources to help them care for their aging family member. They should closely examine their ability to provide long-term care in their home. They should avoid offering personal home care unless they thoroughly understand the demands and expenses involved. They need to avoid over-extending themselves and should not expect problems to disappear once the elderly person moves into their house.

As EMS providers, we routinely treat elderly patients. This situation won't change anytime soon. Elder abuse is a crime, and as the so-called "gatekeepers" in the new health-care landscape, we need to be as vigilant in recognizing elder abuse as we are in recognizing and reporting abuse in children, spouses or any other victims we interact with.

References

1. Kaudner D, Schwab W: "Trauma in the elderly."
   Emergency Magazine. 23(2):22, 1991.
2. Rose C, editor: "Emergency care of the elderly."
   Emergency Medical Clinics of North America.
   May 1990.
3. Ibid.
4. Administration on Aging: The National Elder
   Abuse Incidence Study; Final Report. September
   1998.
5. Ibid.
6. Ibid.
7. Rose
8. Ibid.

When Trauma Masks a Medical Emergency

"Education is an admirable thing, but it is well worth it to remember from time to time that nothing that is worth knowing can be taught."—Oscar Wilde, Intentions

What connotations does the word *suspicious* have? For most, the word carries a negative association. The media is full of suspicious types, from TV shows about detectives to the old *Mission: Impossible* shows in which the Border Patrol asks for the character's identity with predictable results. Can being suspicious ever be a good trait?

Let's examine this case to see if this EMS crew was suspicious enough.

Scenario

This sunny day finds you working with your regular partner. The radio suddenly squawks, "43 X-ray for motorcycle MVA, in front of the cemetery at the intersection of Woodhaven Blvd. and Metropolitan Ave. Time out is 1139." Nice, you think, a motorcycle down in front of a cemetery—how convenient for the rider.

As you move through traffic, you think of all the possible motorcycle accident permutations. They're the trauma equivalent of a sick call: the severity could range from no injuries to traumatic arrest and anything in between. You never quite know what you're getting yourself into.

You arrive on scene to find a motorcycle on its side. Your patients are an elderly husband and wife dressed in leather riding outfits. You and your partner each take a patient.

You approach the wife. She's 64 years old and has bilateral, open fractures of the lower legs. The bone ends have ripped through her pants—a dramatic injury, but with only a small amount of visible bleeding.

Both patients were wearing helmets, and both remain conscious and alert. The wife says a car struck their motorcycle at the intersection. She has no other complaints, and your examination confirms no other injuries. She takes no medications and has no pertinent medical history. *Her vitals:* pulse 104, respiratory rate 20 and blood pressure 140/88. Her pupils are equal and reactive.

Your partner's patient, a 67-year-old male, complains of flank and back pain that radiates to his groin, along with some abdominal tenderness. He claims to have had most of these pains for the past week or so. He also has abrasions on his right hand, elbow, cheek and chin. He has no other complaints or physical signs of trauma. He doesn't see a doctor regularly, takes no medications and claims never to need either because he's never sick. He denies chest pain or shortness of breath. His chest is intact and shows no sign of injury. *His vitals:* pulse 100, respirations 22 and blood pressure 160/96. You and your partner agree to transport the wife to St. Carolyn's Trauma Center, and the newly arrived BLS crew will follow after immobilizing the husband on a longboard. You present the patient to the ED after a 12-minute transport.

While cleaning your unit, you hear the BLS crew over the radio requesting a trauma alert for the husband. You grab your partner and tell him what you heard. When the husband arrives, ED staff members take over CPR, establish an IV and insert an endotracheal tube. The surgical team notices the patient has an ECG but no pulse. They open the patient's chest, and blood cascades out the thorax. After an hour of unsuccessful surgical machinations, the patient is pronounced dead.

Later, the surgeon asks why you didn't transport the husband first. He listens to your detailed description and rationale, but he doesn't understand your reasoning. An elderly patient plus collision plus belly pain equals an unstable patient. Always.

He also informs you that flank pain radiating to the groin, abdominal tenderness and back pain are the classic presentation of an abdominal aortic aneurysm (AAA). He adds that AAA occurs more often in men than women and is associated with a history of hypertension. You knew this guy had been in pain for several days before the accident; the patient told you that. If you had paid attention to his more subtle signs, symptoms and complaints, the surgeon goes on, this guy could've been rapidly transported and perhaps arrived at the ED salvageable.

Conclusion
Suspicion is an important trait for EMS practitioners to

embrace. In order to look beyond the obvious in EMS, you must develop a suspicious nature that will allow you to critically evaluate all the tip-offs to your patient's conditions and injuries. If you don't turn a critical eye toward an injury or pattern of injuries, errors can occur.

How do you "read" your patients for injuries and sniff out symptoms that aren't obvious? The answer is simple. You need to remain suspicious and search for them on every call.

'Magic' Numbers

"That which deceives us and does us harm,
also undeceives us and does us good."
—*Joseph Roux*, Meditations of a Parish Priest

Can we use numbers to define certain conditions? Sure!
Example: tachycardia—a heart rate greater than 100. In
the field, we find numbers instructive and useful. My
students know that scoring less than 75% on a test or
quiz means they'll need to retest. They also know that
different tests carry different passing scores. Can we find
similar examples of these variable norms in patient care?

Scenario
Your ambulance is activated for a collision on the interstate. It takes approximately 10 minutes to arrive on
scene. You find a two-car, front-end collision with four
patients. Two occupants of one car walk about the scene.
They tell you they're not injured; they're alert and ori-

ented x 3.

A BLS ambulance arrives and assumes care of the two walking wounded. A man in his late 60s sits in the other car. He complains of abdominal and chest discomfort. He wasn't wearing a seatbelt, and the steering wheel is slightly bent. As your partner places the man on high-flow oxygen, you examine him. You find his pupils equal and reactive, neck normal and his chest and abdomen without bruising. The patient is alert and oriented x 3 and tells you he has a history of hypertension and takes propranolol twice a day. He also tells you he has no history of heart disease, asthma or chronic obstructive pulmonary disease.

A police sergeant tells you about a helicopter en route, should you decide to have the patient airlifted to the trauma center 40 miles away. *The vital signs:* BP 110/70, pulse 88, respirations 18. The man's skin is normal—not pale or cool. After conferring with your partner, you decide that the patient is relatively stable and does not need the helicopter. After all, every parameter of perfusion (or shock) is normal in this patient.

Within 10 minutes, the two of you have applied a cervical collar and immobilized the patient to the Kendrick extrication device. Once you move the patient to the ambulance, you tell your partner to hold off on proceeding to the hospital until you start an IV. All the while, the clock keeps ticking.

After several minutes, you've placed the IV and are underway. While en route to the community hospital 10 miles away, the patient tells you that he feels dizzy and passes out. As you rush to take a blood pressure, you find the pulse is gone and the patient is apneic. Because you are the only person attending the patient, you now have the unenviable task of intubating, ventilating and performing compressions on him in the back of a moving ambulance. Man, what you wouldn't give for that chopper right now!

Discussion

What specific learning points can we acquire here? First, thinking that hypotension and tachycardia are absolutes will get you nowhere. Clearly, they aren't. This patient was elderly and taking a beta blocker. The elderly do not respond to the stress of blood loss the way we might expect: they may not have the ability to raise their heart rate in response to stress, even if the patient does not take beta blockers. You can't expect to see that reliable parameter of shock we call tachycardia in an elderly patient.

Also, the patient was not hypotensive by classical interpretation. His BP was 110/70. Is this patient hypotensive? He may in fact be hypotensive if his normal blood pressure is 170/84! This brings us to another myth that we need to destroy. Hypotension is not a blood pressure of less than 90 systolic. Blood pressure is relative and can't be dealt with as an absolute number. Consider any elderly trauma patient with a blood pressure below 120 systolic as hypovolemic until proven otherwise.

On assessment, we also noticed that this patient did not have the pale, cool skin that we expect to see in shock. The elderly have poor response to the messengers in their bodies that compensate for blood loss. This means you may not see the pale, cool skin you have come to expect in shock.

Well, now that we have shot to hell all of the quickly assessed, rapidly measured parameters of shock, how do we assess injured elderly folks? *The magic words:*

mechanism of injury. If the patient could or should be in shock from the injuries suffered in the MVA or fall, you must assume that to be the case and then triage and treat accordingly.

Can we always use numbers to define certain conditions? No, as this month's case illustrates.

7
NEUROLOGICAL EMERGENCIES

Headache Calls

"PAIN n. An uncomfortable frame of mind that may have a physical basis in something that is done to the body or may be purely mental, being caused by the good fortune of another."—Ambrose Bierce,
The Devil's Dictionary

The other day, as my two daughters bickered incessantly, I reached for the bottle of Tylenol. As I did, I wondered, "Is this simply a tension headache? Could it be a migraine or perhaps some other differential diagnosis too horrible to contemplate?" The list of possibilities that I give my students immediately came to mind: encephalitis, hypertensive crisis, meningitis, hemorrhagic stroke, transient ischemic attack or a tumor. (I could almost hear Arnold Schwarzenegger saying, "It's not a toomah.")

As the pain subsided, I thought of how many patients present with headache and other complaints that individually don't add up to much of an emergency, but when considered together may present a totally different picture. Let's examine this case for a demonstration.

Scenario—When 2 aspirin aren't enough

You arrive at work to find you'll be working with Ari Minardos. The dispatcher calls you for a "37-year-old female, sick; 636 Brooklyn Ave., Apt. 6C, between Fenimore St. and Rutland Road. Time out 1502."

While responding to the location, you try to determine why you've been sent to a "sick" call. You review the assignment on the computer terminal: The 37-year-old patient is complaining of a severe headache, nausea, vomiting, neck and leg pain.

You arrive at the address at the same time as a BLS unit, which volunteers to back you up. You enter the apartment and find the patient in a darkened room. According to the patient's husband, the light makes her headache worse. He says she's nauseous and has vomited several times, but has been in good health with no medical history and no medications.

The patient is conscious and able to answer your questions. She complains of a terrible headache that's lasted for the past 24 hours. She has a stiff neck and pain in the lower back and legs. She says she's never experienced a headache this severe. She moves all extremities, but has some weakness on her left side. She does not have a fever; her pulse is 104, respirations are 18; and blood pressure is 150/90.

You place the patient on high-flow oxygen and obtain an ECG. It shows sinus tachycardia with no ectopy. Your partner is tempted to hand off the sick-call patient to the BLS crew, but you object. Although the patient does not have a fever, you suspect meningitis or some other spinal irritation. You move the patient to your ambulance and begin transport to the hospital, 20 minutes away.

En route, the patient becomes less alert. You insert an oral airway and ventilate her with a bag-valve mask. Her pulse remains the same, and you conclude that because she tolerated an oropharyngeal airway, she's a candidate for an ET tube. You place the tube and transport the patient without further incident.

Later, your medical director says you did a great job treating the patient. He reports that she had suffered a subarachnoid hemorrhage (SAH).

Approximately 27,000 cases of SAH occur annually in the United States. The incidence is higher in women than in men. Ten to 15% of SAH patients die before reaching the ED, and 50% die within the first six months, even with treatment. Classic complaints include neck and back pain, photophobia (an abnormal reaction to light), nausea, vomiting and severe headache.

Often the patient will tell you that it's the "worst headache of my life." In the acute phase, seizures occur in 25% of cases. Lateralizing signs (one-sided weakness) present in 60% of cases.

Examine the whole patient
Here's a perfect illustration of a patient who presents with several complaints that taken individually appear benign. However, when examined together, the complaints add up to a catastrophic problem in patient care. Headache calls can take many forms. They can be:

1. Just a headache;
2. A serious problem with headache appearing as just one of several symptoms; or
3. A call that will give you a headache if you don't handle it properly.

Should this surprise us? No. The trauma patient with a fractured arm is a minor injury, but the patient with several fractures may be considered a multi-trauma victim. The same analogy should follow in the medical cases we see.

Headache alone may be a minor issue, but when added to nausea, vomiting and neck pain, the simple headache takes on an ominous overtone. Listen to your patients. Their symptoms often beg to be heard.

Trust Your Instincts

*"And I looked, and behold, a pale horse: and his name
that sat on him was Death ..."—Revelation 6:8*

How should we deal with the patient whose death is not
only imminent, but expected? During our education, we
are told that death is the enemy, that we must do battle
with the grim reaper and regularly cheat him out of his
reward.

We are now regularly instructed about the concept
of dying with dignity, living wills and health-care prox-
ies. Most of us find this legal prattle confusing. How are
we expected to play a game where the rules are constantly changing and the stakes are the well-being and,
sometimes, the life of a patient? Seems like a loaded
question.

Are there any reliable footholds on this slippery
slope of the care of the dying patient? The reassuring
answer is yes, as this case illustrates.

Scenario

The crew was dispatched for a report of an adult female with difficulty breathing. On scene, they found a 55-year-old, peripherally cyanotic female who had been unresponsive to verbal stimuli for 20 minutes. Her family told the crew that the patient has had bone cancer for three years and is in constant pain. The family also said that the patient did not wish to have any heroic measures used to revive her; they want to honor her request but agree to allow an examination.

The crew found the patient had the following vital signs: BP 116/60; HR 122, weak; respiratory rate 6, shallow; CR 2 seconds; and her pupils pinpoint. The family produced the patient's only medication, which was methadone (7 mg, taken orally, every three to four hours for pain). This medication had been prescribed by the patient's oncologist.

How do this patient's symptoms add up for you? It looked like a narcotic overdose—the pinned pupils and hypoventilation, in particular—not end-stage cancer to the crew. The crew examined the medication, trying to rule out an overdose. The prescription was new and almost all the medication was accounted for. The family insisted that the patient took her medication as directed and was in good spirits prior to this event; they again expressed their wish to have the patient die with some degree of dignity.

Unconvinced that this was the presentation of an end-stage cancer patient, the crew pressed for more information. Are there other medications, a medical history or procedures, they asked. The patient's husband, who had been weeping in another room, came in to tell the crew that the patient had gone to the dentist the day before for a tooth extraction.

The man said that about two hours before the incident, his wife had had some tooth pain and had taken a pain pill that had been prescribed by her dentist. The husband produced the prescription: Tylox (5 mg, to be taken every six hours) for pain. The paramedics realized that the dentist had never consulted with the oncologist on pain medications. This is the part of the puzzle the crew had been looking for. Tylox is a combination of the powerful narcotic analgesic oxycodone and Tylenol. The patient had looked like a narcotic overdose to the crew because she was a narcotic overdose!

The crew convinced the family that this was a reversible condition, not the expected end of the patient's life. The family agreed to allow treatment. The patient was ventilated; an IV was started; and naloxone was administered. The patient became pink and responsive. The crew transported her to the hospital.

What is the pearl to be harvested here? Trust your intuition. Most of us, at any level, have well-developed intuition. It is an educator's job to harness and nurture intuition, and the practitioner's job to trust it.

Think about it: Most of us are well aware of what we are doing when we act against our better judgment and doubts. We must learn to trust that plaintive voice called a conscience, which will help us do the best for our patients and ourselves.

This patient made an uneventful recovery from her accidental overdose and went on to live for another two years, for which she was grateful. You see, she got to see a son graduate from college and a granddaughter born. Things are not always what they first appear to be and, as practitioners, it's our job to sift clues to arrive at the correct conclusion. We must learn to trust our instincts.

Assume Nothing

"Mistakes are the great educator, when one is honest enough to admit them and willing to learn from them."
—*Anonymous*

Have you ever looked at a patient and made a decision on their condition based on prejudice instead of knowledge? Let's face it—we all have. And although such action is fraught with danger, no profession remains immune to it.

The following fictitious conversation between a U.S. Naval ship and Canadian authorities off the Newfoundland coast illustrates the danger of making assumptions:

Canadians: Please divert your course 15° south to avoid a collision.

Americans: Recommend you divert your course 15° to the north to avoid a collision.

Canadians: Negative. You will have to divert your course 15° south to avoid a collision.

Americans: This is the Captain of a U.S. Navy warship. I say again, divert your course.

Canadians: No. I say again, you divert your course.

Americans: This is the aircraft carrier U.S.S. Lincoln, the second largest ship in the United States Atlantic fleet. We are accompanied by three destroyers, three cruisers and numerous support vessels. I demand that you change your course 15° north. I say, again, that is one five degrees north, or countermeasures will be undertaken to ensure the safety of this ship.

Canadians: This is a lighthouse. Your call.

(The New York Times 7/5/98)

All of us make assumptions—in our personal lives and on the job. Most of the time, we base these assumptions on experience and fact. Usually, they prove true. However, we sometimes get burned when we base our conclusions on bias. This month's case illustrates how bias interferes with prehospital care.

Your ambulance is dispatched to an unconscious male in an area of town noted for high crime and drugs. Your partner says he wouldn't be surprised if it were another "methadonian" overdose. This thought had already crossed your mind.

Scenario

You arrive on scene, and the surroundings appear safe. You find a 40-year-old unconscious male, lying on the street. His friend, standing next to him, informs you that the man was talking "funny" and then passed out. He also tells you that the patient drinks, but apparently does not use recreational drugs. You find the patient warm and unresponsive to verbal stimuli. His airway remains open. His respiratory rate is 15, but so wildly irregular that you have to count it for a full minute. Sometimes he breathes deeply, other times shallowly with periods of apnea. His heart rate is 100; BP is 140/90.

Your partner reports that the patient has pinpoint, minimally reactive pupils. Your partner says that clinches it as an opiate overdose. As you start the IV, the patient's arms start to flex toward his chest. Your partner holds them down as the IV is started. Per standing orders, you give the patient naloxone. In your experience, naloxone usually wakes up addicts within a minute. But that doesn't seem to happen now. Convinced that this patient has OD'd, you remain on scene 15 more minutes, administering more naloxone, supplemented with thiamine and dextrose. You wait for it to work.

When the patient turns blue and becomes apneic, you and your partner transport the patient rapidly to the hospital, confused about why your treatment hasn't worked. Soon after beginning care in the ED, the physician tells you the patient's problem did not relate to drugs at all. His pinpoint pupils, decorticate posturing, fever and abnormal respiratory patterns indicate an intracerebral bleed at the pons. These patients have a high mortality rate. You realize that he had all the signs, you just didn't see them.

Sometimes, we're so convinced that our conclusions are correct that we don't see what's really going on. Usually this occurs in the heat of battle or other high-stress time. In EMS, this can also occur when we reach conclusions with inadequate information or preconceived ideas. Patients usually can't give us every bit of information necessary for a complete history. But reaching conclusions about patients before arriving on scene usually comprises the first serious error. However, selectively processing information to prove the flawed conclusion is the second—and more serious—error. In

EMS, our job is to notice things in people, especially abnormal things. Do not allow bias and predetermina-tion to blind you—or you'll hit the lighthouse.

8
TOXICOLOGICAL
EMERGENCIES

Suspicion—An Important EMS Asset

"Nothing is easier than self-deceit. For what each man wishes, that he also believes to be true."
—*Demosthenes*, Third Olynthiac

What is the most dangerous place in the world? Is it an infectious disease storehouse or a commercial fishing boat off the coast of Alaska? I think it's under your kitchen sink. On my last inspection of that area in my house, I found no less than two metal cleaners, dishwasher detergent, Drano and some spray that kills fleas on pets—all lethal poisons in their own right. Poisons can ruin your day faster than a bad round of golf. Clearly, homes harbor agents that can subtly manifest themselves in deadly ways. Let's examine this case for an example.

Scenario
On an otherwise quiet day, dispatch sends you and your partner to a call for an "Adult male vomiting. 325

Michael Lane off Rubin Blvd. *Time out:* 1310." Splendid, you think. Why are we tying up an ALS unit on this call? Where are the BLS units? As you arrive on scene, you're directed to the rear of the house and discover why your ALS crew was called—an unresponsive elderly man actively vomiting in the middle of his garden.

As you immobilize the patient's C-spine, begin suction and prepare him for intubation, your partner obtains a quick history. The patient's wife explains he had a bypass operation several years ago and has a weak heart. He takes digoxin, Lasix and Slow-K. He went out to the garden an hour ago, and when she called him in for lunch, he didn't answer. She found him and called 9-1-1.

Your partner tells you the patient is incontinent and has diarrhea. You notice the patient's pupils are constricted and his eyes are tearing profusely. The patient's heart rate is 45. At this point, your patient becomes apneic and cyanotic. You successfully intubate him with his head in a neutral position and begin bagging him. The patient has some wheezes in his lung fields, and the end-tidal CO_2 detector indicates your tube is in the trachea.

The ECG demonstrates sinus bradycardia at a rate of 45. Blood pressure is 80/46, and you obtain venous access. You start the IV in the right antecubital and administer saline solution.

Your back-up BLS unit arrives and finds an empty bottle near the patient in the tomato plants—a bottle of Malathion. They also find the sprayer he was using. You and your partner correctly decide the patient is likely experiencing organophosphate poisoning and normal poisoning treatment won't be effective. You call medical control and present the patient condition to the doctor.

The doctor agrees the patient has all the symptoms for organophosphate poisoning. You learned to remember these symptoms with the acronym SLUDGE: salivation, lacrimation (excessive tearing), urination, diaphoresis, gastrointestinal motility and emesis. The medical command physician orders 2 mg atropine via IV bolus and asks you to monitor the patient, repeating the dose every 20 minutes until the symptoms disappear.

You begin transport to the receiving hospital. The transport proves uneventful, and the patient improves somewhat after you repeat the atropine dose during the ride.

In the hospital, the physician administers another antidote for this particular poisoning, pralidoxime (Protopam). He explains it activates cholinesterase, an enzyme that reverses the poison's effects.

Discussion
You check back on the patient later in the week and learn he had a smooth recovery and was discharged after a few days. A week after his discharge, he and his wife stop by your station to drop off several pounds of tomatoes from their garden as a thank-you gesture. (They've washed them, of course.)

Although we tend to think these particular toxidromes occur only on farms in the hinterlands, poisonings can occur in the most urban of settings or in places you might not otherwise suspect. The trick to assessing a poison victim is really no different from that of any other patient. Often, you need to suspect a problem in order to recognize it. A baseball manager once said the most important quality a ballplayer can have is something that can't be coached—speed. I believe the most important quality an EMS provider has is something that can't be taught—suspicion. We can easily teach folks the skills, but it's much harder to make them suspicious.

When Good Isn't Enough

*"Expedients are for the hour, but
principles are for the ages."*
—Rev. Henry Ward Beecher,
Proverbs from Plymouth Pulpit, 1887

Ever had someone leave a job unfinished? The carpenter
who begins remodeling your house and never finishes it or
the electrician who begins re-wiring and doesn't complete
the job. Annoying isn't it? Sure—especially if you're the
unfortunate soul who is inconvenienced by them.

It's important to remember that these irritations don't
begin to compare with the consequences suffered when
people in other occupations don't finish their jobs. Notable
examples include: the baggage handler who doesn't properly secure the cargo door on an aircraft, which results in
a crash with great loss of life; or the mechanic who doesn't
tighten the lug nuts on a wheel, which causes it to fall off
on the highway. Newspapers are filled with stories of people and agencies that don't properly discharge their

responsibilities—usually with unfortunate consequences. What does this have to do with EMS? Let's examine this case to find out.

Scenario

You're a part-time medic working with a seasoned, full-time partner in a busy system. The day has been quiet: You've actually completed the Sunday crossword puzzle in record time. While driving around your primary response area, your partner starts a lively discussion on the relative merits of several paramedic programs in your region. As you extol the virtues of your program, you receive an assignment for an "adult male, overdose, on the elevated train platform, Benjamin Blvd. and Alan Avenue station."

Your partner mutters in disgust as you drive to the assignment. On arrival, you hump equipment up the station stairs to find a 30-year-old male, unconscious with central cyanosis and pinpoint pupils. His respirations are 5, and his heart rate is 105. "Great," your partner says, "another narcotic smurf."

The patient's friend tells you that the patient has been taking Darvon Compound for the last hour and then finally passed out on the platform. As you write this down, you see your partner rolling up the patient's sleeve and placing a tourniquet on his arm. She draws 2 mg of naloxone from an ampule and injects it into the patient's upper arm muscle. She then draws more naloxone and injects it directly into a vein in the antecubital area.

You're uncomfortable because this technique wasn't taught in your program. As you begin to question your partner, the patient sneezes and wakes up. You ask him what he took, and he tells you he "didn't take nuthin." There's a surprise: This guy was reanimated with naloxone, but he didn't really overdose on an opiate (yeah, right).

You realize that the patient's "I didn't take nuthin" is the equivalent of the drunk's "I had two beers." While you ponder the analogy, the guy pushes you aside and walks down the platform. Your partner tells the cops to write up the paperwork as "a drunk sent on his way," and she gathers her equipment together. Once again, you're uncomfortable with this, but what can you do? After all, you're just a part-timer.

An hour later, you're still pondering your partner's actions and your own inaction. As you begin to discuss it with your partner, the dispatcher sends your facility's BLS unit to a "major trauma, man under a train ... Benjamin Blvd. and Alan Ave." Your partner pales and your palms dampen as you respond as back up. They arrive first and notify dispatch that they have an obvious DOA. You arrive and find that it's the same patient that your partner "hot-shotted" earlier. Your palms are clammier now as you wonder how things can go so wrong so quickly.

Worth doing well
As children, our parents told us not to start anything we couldn't finish. We were also told that things worth doing were worth doing well. Somewhere along the line these medics forgot those bromides.

Is dealing with addicts and similar individuals the high point in our professional lives? Clearly not, but dealing with them and the related unpleasantness is part of the job. This medic made it too convenient for the addict to get up and "go back to business"—taking and dealing drugs. This patient should have received proper on-scene care (IV started and naloxone titrated up to increase respiratory rate) and been transported to the hospital. Not given just enough care to get him in front of a moving subway train. Make decisions based upon your training—not your tenure.

Routine Calls

"Luck is a mighty queer thing. All you know about it for certain is that it's bound to change."—Bret Harte, "The Outcasts of Poker Flat," 1868

Most of us agree that EMS is exciting. The lack of a routine and the expectation that anything can happen is a definite draw for the profession. Like most of you, I've had numerous forgettable (read: predictable) jobs. I found their boring, unchanging routines stifling. Personally, I could never work in those environments for any length of time.

On the other hand, EMS seemed to lack the predictability that I found so disagreeable. Some other professions don't seem to get boring either. Piloting an aircraft sounds like an exciting and stimulating job, right? I thought so until I spoke to a friend who was a second officer on a DC-10. Because computers tend to do most of the flying, he found his job terribly boring. (OK, one preconceived notion shot to hell.) I've also thought that being a police officer must surely have more than its share of variety and excitement. But for some, the reality is a let down: barking dog complaints at 3 a.m. and frequent domestic disturbances.

Get the picture? Life isn't episodic television. And one thing is clear: Experience demonstrates that EMS is also susceptible to a level of routine and complacency. This case demonstrates the potential dangers of treating things in EMS as routine.

Scenario

You have just stopped to order Chinese food when the dispatcher activates your paramedic unit and a BLS ambulance for a "15-year-old male with chest pain, 1010 Jane Street, cross-street of Sarah Blvd.—in the Elizabeth Apartments." As you respond, you ask your partner how the dispatchers know when you're just about to eat. The two of you agree: they just know, the same way tornadoes know to hit trailer parks.

On arrival you find a 15-year-old male, who has complained of "squeezing" pain for the last 45 minutes. He says the pain is in the center of his chest and doesn't go anywhere. The patient has no shortness of breath or dizziness. He denies any history or medications and tells you that he's in good health and doesn't use recreational drugs.

The BLS unit arrives on scene. The patient's BP is 108/70, his pulse is 120 and respiratory rate 24. In your system, the medics (after evaluating the patient and determining no need for ALS) can release the patient to the BLS unit for transport. In this situation, the EMTs offer to take the patient to the hospital. You and your partner agree. After all, he's just 15 years old—he can't be having a heart attack.

As you move him to the ambulance, he has what appears to be a seizure. You rush to his side as the seizure stops. As you try to rouse him, you realize he's apneic and pulseless. While you bag the boy and the EMTs start compressions, your stunned partner places him on the monitor and tells you that he is fibrillating. You defibrillate him at 200 and 300 joules without result. Finally, at 360 he converts to an acceptable rhythm with a pulse.

As you transport him, he regains consciousness, wondering what happened. He's quickly stabilized and admitted to the medical ICU. A few days later you learn that your patient had a heart attack due to high levels of cocaine in his blood. You and your partner realize luck was in your favor. This situation might have turned out very differently for the patient and your crew had you left the patient in a totally BLS environment.

EMS calls are like snowflakes; from a distance they seem identical. But up close, they are each quite different. Many of us see so many patients that we tend to group them into categories of expected symptoms and outcomes. These expectations tend to be correct a majority of the time, but we always run the risk of getting burned. What prehospital providers do every day is complicated and arduous. But no one pays much attention to that fact until something goes wrong. The more we avoid falling into the abyss of routine, the better it will be for us and our patients.

The Importance of Assessment

"Poisons and medicine are often times the same
substances given with different intents."
—*Sir Samuel Garth*

The most interesting thing I have found about EMS is the variability of patient presentations that we see over the years. An excellent example of this is the differing signs and symptoms a myocardial infarction patient can present with: chest pain, abdominal pain, neck pain, toothache, back and/or arm pain, no pain at all (in certain cases), shortness of breath, fatigue, cold sweats, nausea, vomiting, syncope and—finally—"a feeling of impending doom." The best description I've found for the full range of these symptoms wasn't in some high-level EMT or paramedic textbook. It was in the old, reliable pamphlet distributed when I first took CPR years ago.

In EMS, we are so accustomed to the inconsistency of patient complaints that we expect a certain amount of variation. As we'll see in this case, nowhere is this expectation more problematic than when dealing with a patient who has ingested an unknown substance.

Scenario
One beautiful, summer evening, you're working with your partner of two years, Charlie. Honestly, you still can't fathom why Charlie continues to show up for work. He's verbally abusive to other ambulance crews and acts inappropriately with the paramedic students the two of you occasionally precept. Other crews refuse to have anything to do with him and (by association) you.

Dispatch sends the two of you to an "unknown condition at Tara's Inn, on Route 112. Cross street is Davidson Street. Time out 1916." As you arrive on scene, you're met by a young lady walking her boyfriend to the street. The 29-year-old male looks at the sky, complains of neck cramps and speaks with difficulty. Charlie tells the patient to look at him so he can check the patient's pupils; the patient indicates that he can't. At that point, Charlie whispers under his breath that the patient is either intoxicated or a psycho.

Then Charlie takes the vital signs: pulse 100, BP 136/84 and respirations normal depth at 18. The patient is alert and oriented x 3.

You take the patient's history, and his girlfriend tells you that he has seen his private doctor for persistent nausea and vomiting for about a month. The doctor prescribed compazine two days ago. Since taking it, the patient has felt much better—until now. As you start an IV, you ask Charlie to call medical control because you want to consult with the doctor. Charlie balks, asking how much time you want to waste on this guy. You insist that Charlie must call the doctor.

After the patient presentation, the doctor orders the

administration of a 50 mg IV bolus of diphenhydramine to the patient. Within minutes the patient's symptoms disappear, and the transport to the hospital proves uneventful. After admitting the patient to the hospital, the doctor informs both of you that the patient had a dystonic reaction (impairment of muscle tone, which is usually associated with tricyclic antidepressants) to the compazine. The signs can include facial grimacing and spasms, protrusion of the tongue and arching of the back (in addition to the signs your patient presented). Charlie remains remarkably quiet for the remainder of the shift.

Moral of the story
This case highlights the preoccupation that many of us have in the treatment phase of patient care. It really isn't our fault; it was the way we were trained. In many EMS classrooms, the majority of time and effort is placed on treatment, not on patient assessment. Although we don't hear about many cases of wrong treatment decisions, we do hear about cases of missed assessment and incorrect triaging of patients that result in delayed transport or no transport at all with predictable poor patient outcomes. This might have occurred in our case.

The old adage still applies: Assume the worst, and hope for the best.

Beware of Patients under the Influence

"Drunkenness is temporary suicide: The happiness it brings is merely negative, a momentary cessation of unhappiness." —Bertrand Russell

I saw a T-shirt recently with the message, "I don't have a drinking problem. I drink. I get drunk. I fall down. No problem." Although the intent was humorous, the message misleads. Folks who imbibe too much alcohol are prone to problems and injuries.

The risks—to oneself and others on the road—of driving while intoxicated are well known. Alcoholics are disposed to neurological problems, heart and vessel disease, gastrointestinal and immune system difficulties. In addition, most homicides and one-third of all suicides involve alcohol.

EMS providers face chronic alcohol abusers regularly. These patients often prove difficult to assess and treat. This case illustrates the fact that alcohol's neurological effects can mask many injuries.

Scenario

You're working the 8 a.m. to 4 p.m. shift. Rain has threatened all day. Your shift partner is Gary, a burned-out medic with a bad attitude: He walks all but the sickest patients to the ambulance.

Shortly after the rain begins, the dispatcher calls you for a "collision with personal injuries, Forest Pky. between Flanagan Ave. and Hicks St." Every time it rains, mayhem ensues on Forest Pky., an old, winding, two-lane road under heavy construction.

On arrival, you find a 37-year-old male walking around on scene. He tells you that he was struck by a car. Witnesses confirm that a car, which left the scene, struck the man. As your partner evaluates the patient, you note that the man slurs his words and has a heavy odor of alcohol on his breath.

The patient's vitals are stable, but he complains of severe pain in his leg each time he takes a step. Nevertheless, Gary walks the patient to the ambulance and instructs him to get in. You know this isn't the correct procedure, but the patient was walking on scene and is intoxicated.

The ride to the hospital proves uneventful. As you walk the patient to a bed in the ED, the patient complains that his pain on walking has increased. The doctor gives you a sideways glance when you report the pedestrian vs. auto collision. You go back in service.

The next day, your supervisor and medical director tell you the patient decompensated in the ED and died. An autopsy reveals four pelvic fractures and numerous lacerations to internal organs. A knot forms in your stomach when you anticipate the questions to follow.

Do we commonly see intoxicated patients? Is that a reason to under-treat them? Should the medics have suspected internal damage? You know the answer to these questions.

Assessment complications

The mass media make much about the terrible costs of drug abuse and the violence that ensues from the trade in illicit drugs. However, because of its societal acceptability, alcohol may carry a higher cost.

Early in my EMS career, I learned that intoxicated patients are walking, breathing lawsuits. These range from "two-beer attorneys" to unconscious drunks. We must remain more suspicious than usual in these cases because intoxicated patients generally give us unreliable information.

Assessing the alcoholic patient may be the toughest assignment we face. The assessment picture varies greatly: Patients can be alert, unresponsive or any level in between. The patient may experience slurred speech, blackouts and, at high alcohol concentrations, respiratory depression.

The chronic alcoholic may be malnourished or hypoglycemic with nausea, vomiting and abdominal pain, in an acute poisoning state. Chronic abusers may have actively bleeding esophageal varices. Seizures may be the first manifestations of alcohol withdrawal.

Think about it: Is your patient combative because he has an expanding bleed in his head or because he's consumed too much alcohol? Is he unconscious from acute alcohol poisoning or a stroke?

We can too quickly decide that a patient is just drunk and find it easier to walk them to the ambulance than to properly package them. Such oversights can carry tragic results. The picture varies so much that providers must keep their minds open to the possibility that a patient may have alcohol poisoning. Treat accordingly, and you'll avoid some nasty surprises.

As the Stomach Turns ...

"Mistakes are like knives that either serve us or cut us as
we grasp them by the blade or handle."
—*James Russell Lowell,* Fireside Travels

Most of us—no matter how long we work in EMS—will
always have times when we fight our stomachs. For
some of us, the image of a horribly injured patient causes our stomachs to flip. For others, the smell of a gastrointestinal bleeder does it. The one thing most of us
seem to singularly dislike is the actively vomiting
patient. The sound is not aesthetically engaging, and the
partially digested stomach contents are equally displeas-
ing to the nose and eyes.

For all of the angst we endure when watching a
patient throw up, we learn that—at times—we should
pharmacologically encourage our patients to do so. We
occasionally use syrup of ipecac for overdoses and toxic
ingestions. We're properly cautioned not to cause vomiting in unconscious patients or those who have con-

sumed petroleum products or caustics. Are there other times when we shouldn't administer an emetic? Let's check out this case to find out.

Scenario—OD on secobarbital

One crisp winter day, you're working with Bob. As you check your vehicle together, the conversation turns to talk radio and the need to get news from outside the mainstream media. The dispatcher summons, "Medic 12-Zebra, respond to an overdose, 1245 Lisa Ave., between Keri Street and Michelle Lane. Time out is 0809."

As you drive, your partner looks up the assignment history on the data terminal in your vehicle. According to the caller, the patient consumed an unknown amount of a prescribed sleep medication approximately 10 minutes earlier. As you pull up to the single-family dwelling, a bystander directs you inside to a 30-year-old female patient.

You find the patient alert and oriented to person, place, time and event. She tells you that she took 30 100-mg capsules of secobarbital, which the doctor prescribed to help her sleep. She denies taking anything else. Her pupils are equal and reactive to light. Pulse is 80, respirations 14 and blood pressure 120/80.

The patient has no significant medical history. However, in the course of your exam, she tells you that she has personal difficulties and doesn't want to live anymore.

Your partner places the patient on oxygen and a cardiac monitor. She agrees to treatment and transport. Both you and your partner agree the patient is an appropriate candidate for ipecac. You administer 30 ml of the syrup and have the patient wash it down with three glasses of water. You decide to wait 10 minutes before transporting her to see if the medication works and avoid having to clean up the mess her vomit would create in the back of your ambulance.

As you repeat the vitals and observe the patient, she gets drowsy. Now, you think, would be a good time to transport her to the hospital. As you move her to the ambulance, she appears to fall into a light sleep. Then she begins to retch. You and your partner quickly roll her on her left side to aid in drainage of her stomach contents.

You then place the patient supine to perform endotracheal intubation and protect her airway. As you visualize the glottic opening, the patient vomits again. Again you roll her, hoping she didn't aspirate and trying to forget about the 85–90% mortality associated with aspiration of gastric contents. You suction her aggressively.

When you finally get the patient intubated and listen to her lung fields, you hear ominous, low-pitched noises and gurgles indicative of aspiration. You assist her ventilations with a bag-valve mask as you make the 12-minute trip to the hospital.

You find out later that day that the patient was admitted to the medical intensive care unit on a ventilator. She aspirated vomit prior to the time you inserted the tube in her trachea. A week goes by before the medical director calls you in to discuss the situation. The patient has regained consciousness, but has significant damage to her lungs. Her prognosis remains grim.

The doctor says you could have easily managed the patient's overdose by transporting her and managing her airway. He says you complicated her condition by administering the ipecac. He points out that several drugs, including secobarbital and certain antidepressants, act rapidly, causing a patient to lose consciousness before Ipecac can begin to work. He recommends you consider giving Ipecac only when you or someone on scene witnesses the overdose.

Do no harm

This patient had not ingested a caustic substance nor a petroleum distillate, and she had a patent airway. You thought you were doing the right thing. However, this case illustrates how even when we treat our patients in good faith and in accordance with our basic training, we can still do harm.

How can we prevent this? Thoroughly educate practitioners to operate in the field and weigh the risks and benefits of all treatment. Also, tell them about the good, the bad and the ugly of what can occur when we treat patients.

9
ENVIRONMENTAL EMERGENCIES

Summer Snafu

Modest doubt is called the beacon of the wise.
—William Shakespeare

Most of us look forward to summer more than any other time of year: barbecue season in high gear, kids out of school and beaches open. Summer also means vacation season. (Unlike many of you, I remember how to go on vacation. I leave the pager on my desk, store the laptop at home and give the family my undivided attention.)

But summer and vacations also bring a particular brand of emergency medical problems. From drownings to heat strokes to bee stings, summer remains one of the busiest times for our business. And working in 90-degree days when you can cut the humidity with a knife makes it tough to think clearly. During summer we may also miss uncommon ailments because they present similarly, as we observe in this case.

Scenario

Your partner for the shift has worked in EMS for the past 20 years. An excellent clinician and mentor to many, Art was your senior instructor in the paramedic program a few years ago. Back then he had quite a reputation as an instructor who didn't put up with much. He had high expectations of his students, which caused many to refer to him as "Ayatollah."

Your truck is dispatched to "Building 269 at the international airport for an adult male with an allergic reaction on an incoming aircraft." As you head to the airport, you remember that assignment information from the airport is usually unreliable. So you're not sure what you're getting into. On arrival, you are directed to the tarmac and onto a large jetliner. Your patient, a 34-year-old, complains of difficulty breathing and has a red rash around his neck. You also notice that he has some edema in the neck region. He claims that this started just after he ate the meal in coach—some mystery fish product.

Now the patient tells you that his fingertips are numb and he feels like something is "boring into my hip joint." As Art puts the guy on oxygen, you obtain vital signs: BP 98/76, pulse 110, ECG shows sinus tachycardia at 110 and respirations 22 and shallow. Lung sounds remain clear despite the patient's insistence that he feels as if he is choking. The abdomen is benign; he has no jugular vein distention; and his pupils are equal and reactive. You detect the smell of alcohol on his breath as he tells you he had a drink about an hour ago. The skin on his extremities appears somewhat edematous.

You feel that treating this guy for anaphylaxis is the way to go because this case seems like a classic example. Art continues interviewing the patient as you start a saline line. Then you overhear the patient telling your partner that he was scuba diving off the outer banks of North Carolina earlier today and then rushed to get the plane home. He dived at 90 feet for about 35 to 40 minutes. He knows that the dive table limits him to 30 minutes at that depth. If he stays down any longer, he needs to stop on ascent or risk decompression sickness. He insists that he has dived to this depth before without a problem, but never with a flight directly afterward.

Art informs you that all modern aircraft maintain cabin pressure equivalent to 5,000 to 8,000 feet and that has caused the patient to experience decompression sickness (the "bends"). The patient had used dive tables set up for a diver to return to sea level, not to quickly go to a higher altitude after a dive. The dissolved nitrogen in his body expanded at the plane's altitude, causing the condition. You and your partner continue treating the patient. This includes high concentration of oxygen, maintaining ventilatory and cardiac function, fluid resuscitation and rapid transport for recompression. You then call the dispatcher to request the nearby specialty center to have their hyperbaric medicine staff ready for your arrival.

As we've learned many times in the past, what looks like an obvious case one moment can change in the blink of an eye to a completely different situation. Our mission is to think on our feet and respond accordingly. Approach each patient and situation with an open mind, and allow your clinical judgment to dictate patient care.

Seasonal EMS Tightrope

"To everything there is a season."—*Ecclesiastes 3:1*

When asked his age during an interview, the late singer, songwriter and activist Harry Chapin once said he was 35 seasons old. He thought about his life in seasons rather than years because he enjoyed the changes each season held for him.

Many of us live in areas where we can enjoy seasonal changes. Where I live in the northeast, we get four distinct seasons. Winter is great for skiing and sledding; summers are great for the beach, boating and swimming. Fall and spring may be the most delightful seasons of all because they're temperate and comfortable.

In EMS, motor-vehicle crashes and many other emergencies have no seasonal propensity. However, some assignments seem to occur more frequently during particular seasons. Let's examine this case for an example.

Scenario

It's a warm day in late August. Your partner Brian, a new paramedic hired straight out of school, is a capable young guy who's worked with you for the past two months.

The two of you receive a call to "the Schwartz Pavilion, for an adult male drowning—time out, 1406." The Schwartz Pavilion is a parking structure at Rowe Beach, a large area frequented in the summer by 50,000–100,000 swimmers, bay rats and revelers.

You fight the beach traffic and arrive at the pavilion to find lifeguards surrounding a 22-year-old male they had pulled semi-conscious from the surf. The patient, Bodie Jones, is now conscious and alert x 3. The lifeguard reports the water is warm, and the patient was submerged for less than two minutes—important factors in submersion cases because submersion time and water temperature factor directly into survival rates.

You obtain the patient's vital signs and place him on high-flow O_2 via nonrebreather mask. His BP is 112/70, pulse 100, respiration is 18 and lung sounds are clear in all fields. The patient denies any medical history, seizures, allergies or recreational drug use. He says he consumed only two beers prior to swimming. (Yeah, right. You silently wonder how anybody ever gets drunk because no one ever drinks more than two beers.)

You place the patient on the cardiac monitor and document a sinus rhythm of 100. The patient insists he doesn't want to go to the hospital, saying he's suffered enough embarrassment today to last a lifetime. First, he complains about being pulled out of the water by the Baywatch gang. Then he squawks about the crowd that gathered after the paramedics arrived on scene. He says going to the hospital in an ambulance would be more than he could tolerate.

You and your partner insist that he go to the hospital for further evaluation. The police arrive and tell him the same. He finally agrees. You establish an IV of normal saline and begin transport. The trip to the hospital proves uneventful, with Bodie asking how long he'll have to wait in the ED. You present your patient to the staff and go back in service.

Delayed reaction
The tour ends. Several days later you attend a required CE session—the emergency medicine/EMS call review. At the end of the review, you and Brian learn that Bodie was in the ED for three hours when he began to experience shortness of breath, cyanosis and altered mental status.

He was intubated in the ED and transferred to the ICU. Two hours later he developed rales, became hypoxic and his O_2 sats plummeted. He then suffered a cardiopulmonary arrest, and the ICU staff couldn't resuscitate him.

As you absorb the shock of your patient's outcome, the medical director says your decision to insist on Bodie's transport was judicious. On scene, near-drowning patients often appear symptom-free and try to refuse treatment. However, many near-drownings result in delayed aspiration pneumonia or respiratory distress syndrome and subsequent respiratory failure. These complications can occur as long as 24 hours following submersion. Therefore, all near-drowning cases need to be seen in the ED.

This information does little to comfort you. You never even entertained the possibility that your patient might not survive. Some patients die. That's part and parcel of an EMS career. But this case causes you to go home, speak to your spouse at length about it and lose more sleep than normal after a bad call.

The National Safety Council reports drowning as the fifth leading cause of accidental death in the United States—responsible for more than 4,500 deaths per year. Also, 80,000 near-drowning incidents are reported each year.

Cases like this one are seasonal—occurring predominantly in the summer. Therefore, keep your EMS senses on high alert for near-drowning cases during the summer months. But regardless of the season, good medical practices and sound patient assessment are necessary year-long as you walk the seasonal EMS tightrope.

Caught Cold

"When anyone asks me how I can best describe my experience in nearly 40 years at sea, I merely say, 'uneventful.' Of course there have been winter gales and storms and fog and the like. But in all my experience, I have never been in an accident ... of any sort worth speaking about. I have seen but one vessel in distress in all my years at sea. I never saw a wreck and never have been wrecked nor was in any sort of predicament that threatened to end in disaster of any sort."
—E.J. Smith, 1907, captain, RMS Titanic

From the beginning of time, humanity has suffered for its nakedness. As creatures of temperate environs and lacking animal fur and the insulating fat layers of seals or whales, we must sheathe ourselves in wool or other fabrics to journey and survive in inhospitably cold climates. Lacking the ability of many animals to shed tremendous amounts of heat, humans feel equally uncomfortable in areas with high temperatures and humidity. If we shed layers of clothing in these environments in exchange for the cooling process, our skin burns and blisters.

A fair amount of technological effort has gone into keeping us warm in winter and cool in summer. In EMS, a patient's response to cold or heat has always caused concern. Although we can expect an Everest climber to suffer hypothermia or a jungle explorer to have a heat stroke, patients in the environments where most of us work may have a more obscure presentation. Let's examine this case for an example.

Scenario
The temperature is in the low 50s, and the downtown area maintains its frenetic Saturday night pace. You imagined urban EMS like this when you sweated your butt off on cardiology in the paramedic program. The dispatcher's disembodied voice announces, "Man down in the street in front of Jeff's Tavern, at the intersection of Clyde and Payne Street. Time out 2010."

Outstanding. Another intoxicated Saturday night partyer. As you arrive on scene, you observe a 55-year-old male, unsteady on his feet and markedly slurred in his speech. The police say bystanders claim the man never fell, but was seen walking erratically and speaking incoherently. He shows no signs of trauma.

Your well-practiced nose detects the aroma of inexpensive alcohol. He answers most of your questions regarding his chief complaint, history of present illness, medications, medical history and previous hospitalizations by answering, "No thanks. I don't smoke." He's clearly intoxicated and becomes more delirious by the minute. You and your partner decide to transport him to the city hospital 30 minutes away, where he can sleep it off in their special sobriety unit.

You sit on the squad bench and begin filling out the paperwork. You plan to take his vitals before you get to the hospital—but after the paperwork. You notice your partner seems to hit every pothole in the city.

Your patient suddenly seizes and becomes apneic. As you ventilate him, you can't feel a pulse on his cold skin. You scream for your partner to divert to the nearest hospital—thankfully, only a block away.

The ED staff place the patient in the resuscitation bay and go to work. They place a thermometer probe in the patient's esophagus. It indicates the patient's temperature as 30° C, or 86° F. Your stomach twists as you realize you would have recognized the patient's hypothermia, aggressively treated it and transported the patient to the nearest hospital had you only taken his vitals or touched his skin prior to ventilating him. How are you going to explain why you didn't take his vitals?

Conclusion
Lucky for you, the staff rewarm and resuscitate your patient. Once again, preconceived notions and nonadherence to routine have turned a relatively benign situation into a life-threatening one for the patient and a career-threatening one for the EMS provider.

People with alcohol on their breath beckon us to look beyond the obvious. Hypothermia can mimic a stroke and, in severe cases, induce a coma. Delirium, slowed reflexes, vision and speech problems also commonly occur. In the urban setting, illicit drug use and overdose, alcohol abuse, psychiatric emergencies and major trauma are all associated with hypothermia.

Don't wait for the weather to mimic Duluth, Minn., or Fairbanks, Alaska, to suspect hypothermia. Factors other than severe weather and extreme temperatures can precipitate hypothermia.

When patients present with hypothermia, warm them and handle them gently. Hypothermic hearts are irritable and will fibrillate if your patient gets bounced around or treated roughly. *The important thing:* Recognize your patient is cold, notwithstanding other distractions. Avoid biases and diversions. Perform vitals before paperwork, and use the thorough and discerning eye and suspicious nature inherent in most, if not all, EMS providers.

The Most Important Piece of PPE

"Half the modern drugs could well be thrown out the window, except that the birds might eat them."
—Martin Henry Fischer (1879–1962)

We have been led to believe that some medications do not have any real appreciable downside for patients who receive them. Years ago, how could we imagine that 50% dextrose could be bad for anyone? It is a great "brain-saving" medication for patients who are hypoglycemic with altered mental status. Who would have imagined it might not be good for patients with the same altered mental status caused by bleeding inside their heads? Sure, now we all know that things like isoproterenol, sodium bicarb and calcium chloride probably do more harm than good. Previously, we assumed some medications could be administered with little concern. We now know, however, that they can quickly bite the patient and us in the hindquarters if we're not careful, as this case aptly demonstrates.

Scenario

You and your paramedic partner responded to a report of an unconscious male at a well-known drug location. On arrival, you ascertained that the scene was safe to approach because the police were already present. You found a 30-year-old unconscious patient on the bed in an apartment. Primary survey showed a centrally cyanotic male, breathing at a rate of six breaths per minute. The breathing was of sonorous nature. The patient's pulse was 120 and the BP was 100/70. The pupils were pinpoint. You both noticed a latex tourniquet on the left arm of the patient and a syringe with the needle still in a vein in the forearm. You both realized that you're dealing with an opiate overdose. Seemed like a pretty straightforward assignment.

You put on gloves, goggles and masks and prepared to start an IV. After a few minutes searching for a suitable vein, the infusion was started. As per standing orders, if paramedics strongly suspect an overdose, they can start the IV line, get a glucose level from a glucometer, and administer up to 2.0 mg of naloxone. Once the IV was secured, one of you administered a bolus of 2 mg of naloxone to the patient, and the drug was flushed in. This was the catalyst for an unpleasant turn of events.

About 30 seconds after the naloxone bolus was administered, the patient sneezed twice, opened his eyes and grabbed the syringe and needle that was still in his arm from his own injection. He then poked the bloody needle into your partner's leg. He instinctively pulled the needle out of his leg; the puncture wound was about one inch above the knee. There was what seemed to be about half a cc of the patient's blood in the syringe. The newly combative patient was restrained for the ride to the hospital. Your partner was transported and seen in the ED, where he was referred for counseling, an HIV test and post-exposure prophylaxis as a precaution. He faces years of uncertainty.

Your worst nightmare? Perhaps. Are there positive things to be taken from an unfortunate event? There certainly are! First and foremost, you should have removed the offending syringe and needle from the patient's arm as a function of good medical practice. You and your partner would certainly not have left a knife or a gun in the hand of a patient. Why do so here? What we see here is a failure to don the most important piece of personal protective equipment we own: common sense.

The other error is perhaps not as obvious. It is an error in the administration of the medication—naloxone. Were you allowed to give the 2 mg of the drug? Sure! But did the patient need to receive an amount that completely reversed the respiratory and CNS effects and precipitated violent behavior? I don't think so. Why would you want to have a wide awake, obnoxious IVDA to deal with when you can have a pleasantly sleeping patient who is well-oxygenated and has a respiratory rate of 12/min? Whatever happened to watching your patient as you give the medication to observe for effects, beneficial or otherwise? Just because the protocol says you can give up to 2 mg of a drug doesn't mean that you have to! The choice is up to you.

Don't Become a Legend

"A moment's insight is sometimes
worth a life's experience."
—Oliver Wendell Holmes

Most of us who do this job for very long know that the majority of the time, being an EMS practitioner is a combination of the study of human behavior and detective work. We obtain information and try to make logical and proper medical decisions based on what may be sketchy and incomplete data. After all, we are obtaining this information from patients, not the Library of Congress. Patients, like those of us who attend to them, are human. They make errors or present us with incomplete information. A mentor of mine once said, "You can make mistakes, just don't become a legend!"

One way to avoid becoming a legend is to trust ourselves when we harbor doubts about a patient. And we should also remember that because we are human and make errors, occasionally, we will repeat them.

I have always believed that the difference between adequate and great prehospital practitioners is the ability to make errors only once. This is the beauty of doing this column; it enables folks to gain experience without suffering the pain of making a wrong decision.

Scenario

On the first cold day of the year, your ambulance is sent to a private home. On arrival, you find a 46-year-old female complaining of headache, nausea and vomiting that seem to be abating. The patient has no other complaints. Her only medical history is migraine headaches. She tells you that this felt like a migraine and adds that she often has nausea and vomiting during these episodes. She uses an Imitrex (Sumatriptan) injector to abort the headaches and had used the injector 30 minutes before your arrival.

During the physical exam, you find a seemingly healthy woman with good skin color and turgor, no chest pain or dypsnea and clear lung sounds. The gross neuro exam is unremarkable, and the patient is alert and oriented x 3. Following the exam, the woman told you she felt much better than before and that she would rather not go to the hospital.

The refusal procedure in the city mandates that the crew must call the medical control physician if the crew believes the patient should go to the hospital. The patient has refused transport, but you and your partner ask her once more for the record if she wants to go. She declines and signs the refusal form.

The following morning when you come to work, the night crew tells you they just returned from a DOA female at the same address. Because two police officers investigating the scene had developed headaches, nausea and vomiting, the medics called the fire department. Toxic levels of carbon monoxide were found in the home. Just as you are trying to figure out how to warn your partner about this turn of events, your boss calls you to the office for a conference with the medical director and an attorney.

Well, folks, were errors made? Sure. What were they? Refusals of transport constitute the lion's share of medicolegal exposure. When the public thinks of ambulances, they think of folks being transported to the hospital. To attorneys, a refusal may constitute omission of our most basic duty: taking the patient to the hospital. My concern is with education: Most providers will tell you that a major symptom of CO poisoning is a cherry-red skin color. But these same folks do not readily think of nausea, vomiting and headache as symptoms. It was the way they were educated. In my book, the cherry-red color should go into the same bin as tracheal shift in tension pneumothorax: oft mentioned, seldom seen.

Should this patient have been brought to the hospital? With the benefit of 20/20 hindsight, I can say yes. Would the outcome have been different? Perhaps not. How do we prevent this? The best we can do is learn from our mistakes. Even seasoned EMS folks make mistakes. When I hear that folks have 15 years of experience, part of me wonders if they really have 15 years of EMS experience or one year of experience that they have repeated 15 times. The choice is up to us.

Assessment Hot Potato

*"The gathering of knowledge is the
supreme achievement of man."*
—*Lyndon Baines Johnson, 1964*

Many medical specialties insist on certain things to
make a decision, as discussed recently in one of my
online emergency medicine groups. "Cardiologists want
a thallium scan; allergists want a scratch test; pulmo-
nologists want arterial blood gases; community health
specialists want to see other cases; psychiatrists want to
know about their patient's mother's sex habits," said one
participant.

After that discussion, I wondered what EMS
providers need to make a decision about the care of a
patient. The more I thought about it, the more I realized
that a multi-faceted patient assessment is usually necessary in the field to provide us with enough information
to properly treat our patients. It's what receiving physicians use to judge the quality of our care. Miss the mark,

and a patient sometimes pays the price, as this case demonstrates.

Scenario

It's another hot, humid day in the city. The temperature hovers around 100° F. On days like this, you can't get rid of that wilted, clammy feeling. The air-conditioning in the truck is only a temporary remedy because you'll soon be called to leave your small oasis of cool air for the heat, humidity and sweat of outer environs.

Your partner for this shift, a per-diem paramedic named George, is a city police officer who still works his first love—being a paramedic. He's great fun to work with. As the two of you talk about the pranks others play on him, the dispatcher sends you to an unconscious male at the eighth hole of the Forest Park Golf Course, 101 Forest Park Drive off Woodhaven Boulevard.

As you respond, George questions "why a rational human being would put on those terrible, pastel clothes and play golf on a day like today."

On arrival, you find an unconscious adult male. As it turns out, he's not a golfer but a worker at the course. The patient's airway is open, and he has rapid, shallow respirations of 30. His heart rate is 120. His skin is hot with perfuse sweating. His BP is 88/50. You quickly determine that he has a coma score of 7.

The patient's coworkers report that prior to collapsing he had complained of headache, muscle cramps in his legs and nausea. They told him to drink water, but he couldn't due to the nausea. You begin bagging the patient with 100% oxygen and ask your partner what he thinks. George insists that because the patient is sweaty, it's probably not heat exhaustion. You agree, because the guy doesn't have the hot, dry skin you were taught to look for in heat-stroke patients.

You tube the patient, start an IV and begin transport. Other than bringing him into the air-conditioned ambulance, you and your partner make no attempts to aggressively cool the patient. Then, as you observe some T-wave abnormalities on the electrocardiogram printout, the patient seizes and his pupils become dilated and non-responsive.

One week later ...

At a special review session organized after the patient was determined to be in a "persistent vegetative state," your medical director informs you and your partner that the patient's temperature on arrival at the ED was 106.8° F. The patient was sweaty because he had exertional heat stroke. This occurs in young, healthy individuals who build up heat faster than their bodies dissipate it. Athletes, military recruits and others active in hot, humid environments are most frequently affected.

After the review session, you wish that this discussion had taken place a week prior to the call in question. Would more information on scene have helped? Should this patient have been cooled on scene? This guy was in a coma, tachypneic, tachycardic, had hot skin and was hypotensive. He was practically screaming, "Cool me down!"

Perhaps our two practitioners hung their hats on the oft-repeated adage that "hot-and-dry skin means heat stroke." Maybe they were sick when exertional heat stroke was discussed in class. Or maybe their instructors skipped a discussion of exertional heat stroke altogether.

Remember: Only after we finish our academic programs does our education truly begin. That EMT or paramedic diploma you are so proud of signifies only that you have met some minimum standard. We are charged with learning the rest on the job. Don't wait for a post-incident review session to learn that patient conditions don't always fit an academic mold. Your patient's life depends on your assessment and corrective actions.

Acknowledgments

Writing a book or a monthly column for a magazine often seems like a solitary effort to those who have not had the pleasure. It is anything but. I am indebted to many people who have helped and encouraged me throughout the process. I would like to thank *JEMS* magazine for allowing me the chance to get on a monthly soapbox. Jim Page for your unwavering support over the years. Jeff Berend for listening and making this book happen. The editorial staff, A.J. Heightman, Blaine Dionne, Michelle Garrido, Lisa Dionne for all the polish and work. Keri Losavio, a true gem, for your words of motivation and focus.

Mr. John Becknell, who agreed that a monthly column on case studies from an untested author would be a good idea. Thank you for helping me find my voice.

At Stony Brook, Dean Craig Lehmann, a veteran author, for your encouragement and insight. Dr. Mark Henry for your perspective. Mr. Edward Stapleton, a mentor and friend, for demonstrating and sharing his first-class writing skills.

Mr. Peter Flanagan, for your dedication and commitment to excellence and friendship.

Mr. Arthur Romano, a master teacher, who has been a dear friend and voice of reason for the last 20 years.

Mr. Arthur E. Hoffmann Sr., my late father-in-law. Thanks for your never-ending interest and encouragement. I wish you could see the result.

And all the EMTs, paramedics, readers and students who sent me these cases or commented on them.